# SMART MEDICINE

# SMART MEDICINE

## HOW TO BUY THE PRESCRIPTION DRUGS
## YOU NEED AT A PRICE YOU CAN AFFORD

# PETER WEAVER

Foreword by Richard P. Penna, Pharm.D.,
former head of the American Association
of Colleges of Pharmacy

THOMAS NELSON
*Since 1798*

Published by Rutledge Hill Press, a Division of Thomas Nelson, Inc., P.O. Box 141000, Nashville, Tennessee, 37214.

**Library of Congress Cataloging-in-Publication Data**

Weaver, Peter.
    Smart medicine : how to buy the prescription drugs you need at a price you can afford / Peter Weaver; foreword by Richard P. Penna.
        p. cm.
    Includes index.
    ISBN 1-4016-0139-1 (pbk.)
    1. Drugs—United States—Costs. 2. Consumer education. I. Title.
RS100.W43 2004
338.4'33621782'0973—dc22                                      2004003557

*Printed in the United States of America*

04 05 06 07 08—5 4 3 2 1

*I dedicate this book to Kate Weaver,*
*my wife, my partner, and my inspiration.*

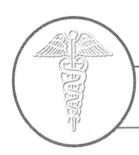

# CONTENTS

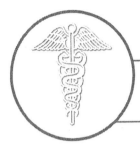

# FOREWORD

Treating diseases with drugs—called pharmacotherapy—is the most frequently used therapeutic practice in health care today. In frequency of use, dollars spent, and acceptability, pharmacotherapy outstrips other forms of therapy such as exercise therapy, psychotherapy, and physical therapy. Its practice includes not only the prescribing of medication by doctors of medicine (physicians) and other authorized prescribers (dentists, podiatrists, nurses, physician assistants, and optometrists), but the use of medication by the vast number of people who treat themselves with over-the-counter (nonprescription) drugs. Many factors have combined to enhance greatly the public's focus on pharmacotherapy. These include:

- The growing number of illnesses that drugs can treat successfully.
- The growing number of potent and effective drugs that are available for public use without prescription.
- The dramatic increase in the promotion of drugs by the pharmaceutical industry, both to the health professions and to the public.
- The spiraling increases in the prices that the public is being asked to pay for prescription medication.

An additional factor, less visible to the public but extremely critical, is the balance between good and harm that accompanies all drug therapy. This balance influences the cost of treating disease. If it tips to the good, the cost declines; if it tips to the harmful side, the costs can be astounding in terms of additional suffering, physician visits, more medication, and hospitalizations. For every dollar that the public spends for prescription and nonprescription medicines, it spends another dollar to correct the harm that these medications can cause.

The use of drugs in treating illness predates recorded history. One can imagine a cave-dwelling early physician or apothecary applying a poultice of leaves and bark to ease the pain of a strained muscle of the community's chief hunter or defender. The later writings of Galen (A.D. 131–201) and Avicinna (A.D. 980–1037) are rich in cataloguing various medicines and mixtures and reveal the importance of medicines in early civilizations. Early on alcohol achieved widespread use not only for its effect on the body but also for its ability to extract the active principles of crude drugs from leaves, barks, and roots into liquid formulations (fluid extracts and tinctures).

Early drugs were from natural origins: plants, animals, or soil. In view of modern-day therapeutics, one might question the effectiveness and safety of many of the early concoctions and mixtures. However, quinine from the cinchona tree, opium and morphine from the opium poppy, belladonna from Jimson weed (and other sources), and digitalis from foxglove ushered into health care truly effective remedies—and at the same time demonstrated the dire consequences of their inappropriate use.

The early pharmaceutical industry in the late nineteenth century introduced the efficient extraction of active drugs from their natural sources and a system of making them widely available to the public through local pharmacies. Moreover, in contrast to the snake-oil salesmen who sold concoctions of questionable efficacy and safety, the pharmaceutical industry in collaboration with the professions of medicine and pharmacy developed important and needed manufacturing, labeling, and potency standards for drugs and the products made from them. These standards continue today and assure the user that the amount of active ingredients stated on the label is actually in the product.

In the twentieth century, the pharmaceutical industry achieved enormous size and stature through its ability to manufacture and distribute medicines efficiently and safely. As World War II was drawing to a close, penicillin became a drug in great demand. Several pharmaceutical companies applied their expertise at fermentation, extraction, formulation, and distribution to make this valuable antibiotic widely available to the wounded men and women who needed it for survival.

Here we are at the beginning of the twenty-first century, and the blush appears to be disappearing from the image of the pharmaceutical industry. On one hand, the industry is responsible for creating and making available a vast armamentarium of drugs to treat an array of illnesses that a few years ago were untreatable (such as HIV/AIDS). Life expectancy has increased steadily due (some say) to the variety of drugs available today. On the other hand, drugs are expensive and becoming more so. Moreover, newer drugs are more potent than the ones they are supposed to replace, which creates hazards to those who use them. Drugs have become very precise, potent, effective, but dangerous tools that, even in the hands of skilled users, have caused and continue to cause costly harm.

It was not long ago that a patient faced with a newly diagnosed illness had no drug treatment available. Today a patient with the same newly diagnosed illness may have a variety of therapeutic options available with a variety of costs and a variety of dangers associated. And herein lies the crux of the problem in modern-day drug therapy. We are awash today in medicines, and great confusion regarding which are the best products to use in any given disease in terms of safety and cost effectiveness. The persuasive promotional tactics of the pharmaceutical industry have enhanced the confusion. Moreover, a given patient may be prescribed drugs by several caregivers and take self-prescribed medicines, which greatly increases the probability of an adverse drug interaction. This has led to very high costs associated with the treatment of diseases: not only costs for the medicines themselves, but also costs associated with the adverse effects caused by the medicines.

Companies that make up the pharmaceutical industry must, as Wall Street corporations, grow financially and show a profit. Consequently, they employ well-trained researchers to create new drugs and marketers to promote these new products to the medical professions and the public. Having made and marketed these new products, they must continue to make and market still newer products to stay competitive and to show a growth in annual profits.

Of course, to make back the increasing costs of research and promotion and show a profit, companies must charge higher prices for each new product they market. The industry has put itself into what some describe as a no-win situation. Their very success depends on creating newer drugs, but newer drugs are costing more and patients are rebelling against paying these higher costs.

This book details pharmaceutical industry practices to induce prescribers and the public to use their latest product and to protect and increase their market share. It also reveals how people may be tempted to save money by pursuing a variety of strategies such as questioning whether a prescription is needed, asking whether a less expensive drug (generic or over-the-counter) might be just as effective, or purchasing drugs through Internet sources or from Mexican or Canadian pharmacies.

The most important message this book conveys is that drug therapy is a complex, costly, and potentially dangerous process. Two costs are associated with drug therapy. The first is the cost of the medicine itself. The second is the cost of getting or not getting well, the cost associated with returning to a productive life or suffering an adverse reaction to the medicine. People who concern themselves with just the costs of the medicine and disregard the dangers of drug therapy do so at their peril.

The bad news is that drug prescriptions are frequently uncoordinated and can be confusing. The good news is that resources are available to assist patients in using their medicine properly. Professional pharmacists are underutilized but very available resources. Not only can pharmacists assist patients in determining potentially less expensive alternative medication, they also can help patients coordinate their drug therapies. While patients may see several physicians who prescribe medication, they should see only one pharmacist, who will maintain a comprehensive medication history and alert physicians and patients to potential problems. Patients should insist that pharmacists perform these services.

The bottom line is that patients must become more active participants in treating their diseases. Active participation means asking questions of physicians and other prescribers. (Is this medicine really needed? What are the side effects? Are there less costly alternatives?) It means that patients must understand fully what their prescribed medicine is intended to do. It means that they must take their medicine as their prescriber indicates. It means that they should utilize available resources to make certain they are well informed. It means bringing their prescribers and pharmacist into the drug therapy decision-making process. It means constant monitoring and continuous questioning.

The important issue here is value. Value balances cost with effectiveness, availability, and risk. This book is about finding value in taking medicines—how to understand, appreciate, seek, and treasure it.

—RICHARD P. PENNA, PHARM.D.

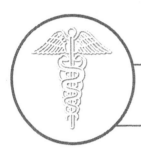

# ACKNOWLEDGMENTS

It took teamwork to get this detailed book done expansively, accurately, and on time. The team spent many hours e-mailing and talking back and forth as new facts were discovered and double checked. I could not have done the job solo.

I am grateful to doctor of pharmacy Richard Penna, who checked the book for medical accuracy and opened up his Rolodex, contacting industry leaders, many of whom he knows personally, to get the latest information.

Editor and researcher Barbara Alpert is a world-class Internet sleuth. She uncovered caches of information involving the latest news clips and technical journal articles to help produce chapters packed with in-depth information.

Over several months, we cast the investigative reporting net far and wide, making hundreds of phone calls and e-mail queries. Here are some of the main contributors: Mark Boesen with the American Health Policy Association; N. Lee Rucker with the National Council on Patient Information; Larry Sasich, Pharm.D., director of Public Citizen; Susan Winkler, director of the American Pharmacists Association; Michael Cohen, Pharm.D., president of the Institute for Safe Medication Practices; Dee Mahan and Judy Waxman with Families USA; David A. Knapp, dean of the University of Maryland School of Pharmacy; internist Kristin A. Thomas, M.D.; and Massachusetts Senator Mark Montigny.

Many others added their voices and ideas to this book, and you will read about them as you go from chapter to chapter.

# PILL POWER

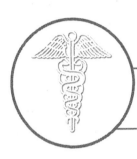

## ONE

## FROM BASEMENTS
## TO BILLIONS

From our earliest recorded history, we know that people sought to understand and control the healing and protective power of medicines. The ancient Egyptians put silver coins in the bottom of their water jugs to kill bacteria and prevent infection. Native American medicine men developed medicinal powders and salves from local plants, the bark of trees, and various minerals; these potions invested them with great tribal authority, especially when they succeeded in healing the sick and saving lives.

In colonial America enterprising doctors and inspired charlatans mixed assorted herbs and mysterious powders into medicines that sometimes worked—and sometimes didn't. Most of the products sold had an alcohol base, which could certainly help persuade the user that the product was a true elixir. Settlers along the northeast coast could buy various remedies and nostrums in local apothecary shops owned and operated by physicians. The doctors usually mixed up their own products, which were often little more than sugary placebos.

The Revolutionary War brought a sudden demand for more powerful drugs that could dull the senses during crude amputations and other battlefield surgeries. Because Philadelphia served as the capital of the new nation, it soon became the center of an emerging pharmaceutical industry. The Philadelphia College of Pharmacy opened in 1821. A year later, a company called Powers & Weightman began manufacturing quinine, which was extracted from cinchona bark and was used to treat malaria.

As Americans pushed farther and farther west, exploring the land beyond the Appalachian Mountains, hucksters operating from wagons produced and sold dozens of "patent medicines." These traveling medicine shows promoted products that were neither patented nor really medicines. Their ingredients were kept secret for good reason, since these "medicines" were little more than alcohol, water, and sugar.

One of the most famous products of the era was Lydia Pinkham's Pink Pills for Pale People. They were supposed to cure the blahs and drive away the blues. Sometimes the pills appeared to work like magic, but this was from the placebo effect—people who believed in the medication sometimes got better simply because they believed they would. The power of suggestion can work wonders. Can the mind convince the body to heal itself? Anecdotal evidence tells us that it's possible.

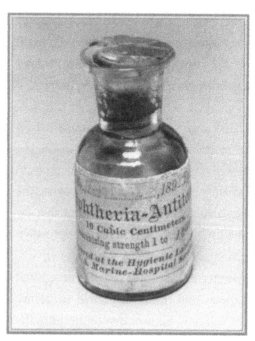

Diptheria antitoxin bottle from the early 1900s

## MILITARY MARKETING

The Civil War produced an extraordinary need for medicines to treat the thousands of wounded soldiers. As battles raged throughout the land, pharmacists, physicians, and businessmen founded the companies that would grow into some of the giants of today. E. R. Squibb & Sons (now Bristol-Myers Squibb Company) and Pfizer started during this period. Eli Lilly, a colonel in the Indiana Artillery, formed Eli Lilly & Company, a pharmaceutical firm that soon became a household name. Pharmacists, such as John Wyeth (the Wyeth Company),

John Dohme (whose company morphed into Merck, Sharpe & Dohme, now just Merck & Company), and Wallace Abbott (Abbott Laboratories) all got their start concocting and producing drugs to meet an urgent military need. Their start-up companies were primarily funded from government coffers.

During the last years of the nineteenth century, most pharmaceutical products were produced by small regional companies, though a few (Eli Lilly and Squibb, among them) had a national presence in the marketplace. It was an exciting time in the industry. Scientists began to discover the causes of diseases as the study of bacteriology led to biological research and new drug formulations. According to a history published by the American Pharmacists Association, among the most important products of the late nineteenth century was antidiphtheria serum, a drug that cured diphtheria, one of the deadly childhood diseases. By 1895 the health departments of major American cities, including New York, St. Louis, and Boston, were producing the serum in their own laboratories.

## How Tragedy Led to Regulation

Disaster struck in 1901, however, when thirteen children in St. Louis died after being given diphtheria antitoxin contaminated with tetanus spores, and in Camden, New Jersey, others developed tetanus after having been inoculated against smallpox. Clearly the government needed to regulate the production and sale of products derived from such dangerous materials. Congress passed the Biologics Control Act of 1902, which President Theodore Roosevelt signed into law. Four years later the Food and Drugs Act would require that all such pharmaceutical products be supervised by the Department of Agriculture. Some of the companies licensed to manufacture these biological products include Parke-Davis, Mulford, and Lederle (named for the director of the New York Health Department, who resigned that position to go into his own lab business).

Legislation over the next decade or so focused on making sure no one made a therapeutic claim for a product that could not be proven. Each new set of regulations further ensured that the American consumer would be as safe as possible when taking a particular drug product. The industry began forming organizations to share information, promote high standards of production, and protect their interests. These included the American Pharmaceutical Manufacturers, founded in 1922, and the Food, Drug and Insecticide Administration (formerly the Bureau of Chemistry, and later shortened to the Food and Drug Administration), founded in 1927.

Just as tragedy forced major changes in the industry years before, another tragedy (the production and sale of an untested "Elixir of Sulfanilamide" that caused the deaths of 107 children and adults) led to the passage of the Food, Drug, and Cosmetic Act of 1938. This new law required manufacturers to prove a product was safe before it could be sold; it also demanded that any drug sold to consumers for self-medication had to be properly and clearly labeled.

## HOW RESEARCH BEGAN
## TO DRIVE THE INDUSTRY

When the twentieth century began, the pharmaceutical industry emphasized manufacturing, not a search for new products. Most companies sold products throughout a particular region, and most new products were speedily duplicated and sold by other companies. But a change was in the wind. Industry leaders looked to the future and realized that continued growth would require developing new products from deliberate research. Instead of depending on other countries for important medications, the United States needed to produce its own.

As part of the World War II effort, companies worked together to develop desperately needed medical products. Two important successes were the production of dried plasma and penicillin. More than 13 million pints of blood collected by the Red Cross were processed into dried plasma for military use. Thirteen pharmaceutical companies (including Abbott, Lederle, Eli Lilly, Parke-Davis, Squibb, Upjohn, and Wyeth) joined forces to process all that plasma. Penicillin was also made possible by extraordinary teamwork. At first, three companies (Merck, Pfizer, and Squibb) led the research, but when six more firms joined in, an astonishing 425 million units were distributed to the military. In 1944 the government asked companies to boost production, and in June 1945, more than 600 billion units were produced, according to the *History of Antibiotics: A Symposium* by John Parascandola.

Once the war ended, research evolved from focusing on diseases caused by organisms to treating "mass market" ailments such as indigestion, arthritis pain, and anxiety attacks. One of the first medicines for stomach disorders, Tagamet, introduced in 1976 by Smith, Kline & French, became the first drug to achieve

## What's in a Name?

Some of the huge pharmaceutical companies we know today got their names from pioneers in medicine and chemistry who were looking for solutions to cope with the primitive ailments of their times. Here are three that have become household names:

**Abbott Laboratories** got its start in 1888, when Wallace C. Abbott, M.D., began making medicines from plants to produce alkaloids for treating stomach disorders and diarrhea. (More than a century later, the company is still studying plant alkaloids in search of new drugs to fight cancer.) During World War II, Abbott helped pioneer the development of penicillin, an antibiotic that saved thousands of American mili-tary lives. In 1952 the company launched erythromycin, an antibiotic that took over where penicillin left off. In the 1990s Abbott developed yet another antibiotic, clarithromycin, to combat germs that had become resistant to erythromycin. Today the company's latest successes include Depakote to treat mental disorders, Lupron for prostate cancer, and Norvir for AIDS. In 2001 Abbott acquired Germany's huge BASF, A.G., a pharmaceutical products manufacturer. The move pushed Abbott several notches higher on the industry's list of companies with multibillion annual sales.

**Merck & Company** was founded in Darmstadt, Germany, in 1658 by Frederich Jacob Merck, owner of the Angel Apothecary Shop. In 1827 scientist Emanual Merck, distant nephew of Frederich Merck, took over and began developing his own chemicals for the apothecary. After World War II, the German company began developing new drugs involving cortisone and hormone preparations. At that point Merck began building a marketing empire that eventually put the company at the top of the industry ladder, with annual revenues of $47 billion.

**Pfizer, Inc.** was founded by Charles Pfizer in 1849 to produce fine chemicals for such items as tartaric acid and cream of tartar for food preservatives. By 1910 annual sales hit $3 million—a huge figure for that era. In 1953 the company developed the antibiotic Tetracyn, and by 1972 Pfizer's annual revenues topped $1 billion. A decade later, a single Pfizer product called Feldene, the largest selling anti-inflammatory medicine, became the first pharmaceutical product to reach $1 billion in annual sales all by itself. In the nineties, Pfizer continued to develop worldwide marketing hits, including Zoloft for depression and Norvasc to control blood pressure. In 1998, Pfizer launched Viagra, a pill designed to treat erectile dysfunction. In a few short weeks, it became an international success, promising anxious males of all ages a chance to reclaim sexual potency.

sales of over $1 billion a year. Those post-war years also saw the launch of such widely used compounds as the antibiotic streptomycin (Merck, 1945) and the first marketed antihistamine, Benadryl (Parke-Davis, 1946).

The industry growth since the advent of World War II has been spectacular. Annual revenue for all the hundreds of pharmaceutical companies doing business at the time was only $150 million. Today, annual revenue for the top nine companies is approaching $200 billion.

## How Marketing Moves Medicine

When today's pharmaceutical companies started in the 1800s, the men who founded them were usually physicians or pharmacists—medical professionals determined to find and sell cures to heal diseases suffered by their patients and customers. In the twentieth century the emphasis changed to manufacturing and distribution. Today the focus of the pharmaceutical industry is on marketing and protecting patents. This trend may be the result of a change in leadership or it may be the cause of it, but pharmaceutical company CEOs today are often recruited from other industries, hired with a mandate to increase profitability, and charged with growing the business by acquisition more than by innovation.

The pharmaceutical industry is certainly not the only one in the U.S. that has changed its focus from making a better product to making a better profit, but it is certainly one of the most successful at it. Critics of the industry accuse it of focusing all its energy on churning up cash, not cures. They point to the practice of tweaking formulas of products that are losing patent protection so the manufacturer can get a new patent or extend the old one and keep on raising prices. The patent is similar to a copyright on a book or CD. It protects the rights to the drug's formula.

## The Challenge of Free Market Pricing

When it comes to pricing a lifesaving drug, how much is fair? Do companies have the right to recover the billions of dollars spent on research and advertising by passing those costs on to the consumer, who's often stuck paying whatever the company chooses to charge?

The answer is not that simple. After years of lobbying, in 1997 the government made it legal for pharmaceutical companies to advertise their products directly to consumers based on the premise that it was educational to the public. So far there has been no successful political movement to reverse this decision. As a result pharmaceutical companies began spending enormous amounts of money on ads hyping their latest drug. They encouraged the public to ask their doctor about the drug, implying that they needed it. Generating a felt need by appealing to the emotions of the consumer, the drug companies created demand. And since many company health plans pay for high-priced prescription drugs, these expensive medications can ultimately end up harming the employees whose out-of-pocket costs are sure to rise. Those costs also play a part in depleting the funds of government programs designed to help people too poor to pay for needed medicine.

Several major studies have fueled this discussion. The Kaiser Family Foundation of Menlo Park, California, found that 30 percent of Americans polled had talked to their doctors about a drug they saw advertised on TV or in a magazine, and 44 percent of those people had received a prescription for the drug upon request. A foundation spokeswoman stated, "More research needs to be done on whether those prescriptions would have been written anyway. Are they actually making people healthier? Were they medically necessary or not?"

In the *Christian Science Monitor* in November 2001, Steven Friday, director of research for the National Institute for Health Care Management in Washington, said, "There is a critical public health issue here, and that's whether it's leading to an increase in inappropriate prescriptions."

The same article quoted clinical studies reported by Blue Cross and Blue Shield, which showed that "95 percent of people diagnosed with arthritis would be fine taking ibuprofen for a few pennies a day. But drug manufacturers are heavily advertising Vioxx for all arthritis patients—a drug that costs a few dollars a day [instead]."

By allowing pharmaceutical companies to spend billions on these ads targeted at consumers, the government contributed, perhaps unwittingly, to skyrocketing costs that put the nation's troubled health-care system at greater risk. And while the industry may insist that the ads encourage consumers to become more involved in their health-care decisions and to seek treatment for many serious illnesses that go un-diagnosed, critics disagreed. Larry Sasich, a pharmacist who heads the consumer-oriented Public Citizen group in Washington, said, "Advertising is not intended to be a benefit to the people it reaches. Its purpose is to increase demand, and it appears to be doing that well."

## HOW HIGH IS TOO HIGH?

So what's too little and what's too much when it comes to setting prices for life-saving or life-enhancing drugs? The Minnesota state attorney general thinks he has a pretty good idea. Mike Hatch filed lawsuits in August 2003 against two drug com-panies for "grossly inflating" the prices of their drugs to treat asthma, bronchitis, emphysema, and other diseases. Bringing suit against Dey, Inc., in Napa, California, and Warrick Pharmaceuticals in Reno, Nevada, Hatch complained that these two companies set unreasonably high prices for their products—charging as much as 800 percent more than the actual cost of producing the drugs.

Why is Hatch taking on these sellers? Because as a result of their pricing, Medicare and Medicaid programs that purchased the drugs were charged millions of dollars more than they should have been, according to Hatch. The suit also alleged that health-care providers prescribed these products to boost their own profits. Other states have filed similar suits against Dey, including West Virginia, Montana, Nevada, Connecticut, and Texas, where the U.S. Department of Justice and the Texas state attorney general reached a multimillion-dollar settlement with Dey on a similar case.

## HOW OTHER COUNTRIES DO IT

Other countries look at drug prices differently. For example, when Norwegian offi-cials look over a new drug for quality approval, they also take a look at the com-pany's pricing data. Limits on what companies can charge are drawn up and become part of the approval process.

Germany, acting as a national purchasing agent for its citizens, puts a lid on what drug companies can charge. The practice is similar to Maine's bulk-purchas-ing initiative (mentioned later) in which it acts as a powerful purchasing agent for its modest-income patients.

In Japan the Special Committee on Drug Prices controls the price of drugs. But according to a Boston Consulting Group report, while Japanese price controls cut prices by more than 60 percent, lower prices and the use of less effective drugs actually raised consumption, thereby increasing citizen drug expenditures by 59 percent.

The question raised in many countries, including the United States, is how to balance the need to encourage research and development by pharmaceutical companies with the need of a nation's citizens for affordable drug products. The future of a private pharmaceutical industry is walking a fine line between a free-market economy and the right of patients to receive lifesaving products.

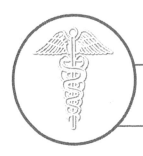

## TWO

## PILL POLITICS

The American pharmaceutical industry has become the biggest, most profitable, and most politically powerful in the world. The top nine companies had sales of more than $166 billion in 2001. These companies spent more than $45 billion on marketing, advertising, and administration compared with $19 billion for research, according to a 2002 study, "Profiting from Pain," done by consumer advocacy group Families USA. And these figures don't tell the entire story. Nobody knows exactly how much the companies other than these top nine make.

If money is power, the pharmaceutical companies have it—and then some. They use this power and the money to shape government policy, to support political candidates, and to manipulate public opinion in their favor. This relentless lobbying effort has one primary goal: to prevent any attempts by the U.S. government to control or limit the prices of prescription medicines.

Some of the effects of aggressive pharmaceutical lobbying are obvious to Americans in every income bracket: health-care costs are rising, insurance rates are sky-high, and the cost of prescription drugs is out of control.

Other effects aren't so easy to spot. These include the ways powerful companies may influence government agencies to streamline the approval process on new drugs or to permit them to limit the public's access to less profitable medicines or lesser-known remedies, by keeping them from going generic.

Then there are the legislative goals of pharmaceutical lobbying—support for laws that benefit corporations at the expense of taxpayers, and action against laws that seek to protect consumers' health and pocketbooks. The "war chests" of major pharmaceutical companies are overflowing with the kind of cash it takes to make an impact on Congress. Who pays the real price for this financial muscle? The millions of American citizens whose daily survival depends on prescription drugs pay the price.

## 2001 Financials for U.S. Corporations Marketing the Top 50 Drugs for Seniors

| Company | Revenue (Net Sales in Millions of Dollars) | Marketing/ Advertising/ Administration | R&D | Profit (Net Income) |
|---|---|---|---|---|
| Merck & Co., Inc. | $47,716 | 13% | 5% | 15% |
| Pfizer, Inc. | $32,259 | 35% | 15% | 24% |
| Bristol-Myers Squibb Company | $19,423 | 27% | 12% | 27% |
| Abbott Laboratories | $16,285 | 23% | 10% | 10% |
| Wyeth | $14,129 | 37% | 13% | 16% |
| Pharmacia Corporation | $13,837 | 44% | 16% | 11% |
| Eli Lilly & Co. | $11,543 | 30% | 19% | 24% |
| Schering-Plough Corporation | $9,802 | 36% | 13% | 20% |
| Allergan, Inc. | $1,685 | 42% | 15% | 13% |
| **Total\*** | **$166,678** | **27%** | **11%** | **18%** |
| (Dollars in Millions) | | $45,413 | $19,076 | $30,599 |

\*Totals may not add due to rounding

From "Profiting from Pain: Where Prescription Drug Dollars Go." © 2002. Courtesy of Families USA and used by permission.

The upward-spiraling costs of prescription drugs may wreak the most damaging effects on those who can least afford it. Seniors, many of whom struggle to survive on limited incomes, often take several prescription drugs every day. Those who suffer from chronic illnesses can't look toward a time when those drugs won't be necessary. And too many older Americans face an impossible task each month—to

## Who Are the Top Nine Drug Companies?

They used to be almost invisible, their names known only to physicians and pharmacists, but then they took their advertising campaigns to the public. Now pages of fine-print drug advertising fill many popular magazines, encouraging readers to ask their doctors to prescribe specific drugs for conditions they have—or believe they might have. While these giant corporations devote large chunks of their marketing budgets to consumer advertising, the cost of these drugs continues to rise. In other words, we're paying twice—once for the advertising to get us to buy the product, and again for the actual cost of purchasing the drug.

| Company | 2001 Revenue |
|---|---|
| Merck & Co | $47.7 billion |
| Pfizer, Inc. | $32.2 billion |
| Bristol-Myers Squibb | $19.4 billion |
| Abbott Laboratories | $16.3 billion |
| Wyeth | $14.1 billion |
| Pharmacia, Corp. | $13.8 billion |
| Eli Lilly & Co. | $11.5 billion |
| Schering Plough Corp. | $9.8 billion |
| Allergan, Inc. | $1.7 billion |
| **Total** | **$166.7 billion** |

From "Profiting from Pain: Where Prescription Drug Dollars Go,"
© 2002. Courtesy of Families USA and used by permission.

make a modest pension or Social Security check cover rent, utilities, groceries, *and* medicine. For our elder citizens and others dependent on medication, "prescription drug poverty" can be a life sentence.

Consider Viola, who is approaching eighty and worked for more than four decades in a shirt factory. Now retired, she's being treated for several chronic illnesses. Each month she spends more than $1,600 on prescription drugs that Medicare doesn't cover. She is increasingly anxious that her modest pension can't keep up with rising drug costs and all the other costs of living. She scrimps where she can, but she's already had to dip into her savings just to pay monthly bills. She rarely eats out, she shops for clothes at thrift stores, and she fears the impact a medical emergency or additional prescription will have on her fragile finances. Under the new Medicare law, which includes a modest prescription drug benefit, Viola can expect some relief but not until 2006. Meanwhile, the law says Viola can purchase a Medicare prescription drug discount card, which could reduce her prescription drug retail costs by 15 percent.

Members of Congress and state legislators are getting a flood of letters and calls from constituents like Viola, who are frightened by the rising cost of their medicines. The Medicare drug benefit will be better than nothing, they say. But for all too many seniors it won't be nearly enough. Millions of Americans do not have health insurance that includes drug coverage. If they do have it at work, it often ends when they retire or are let go.

The big battle to bring down prescription drug costs is taking shape among a growing number of states. The drug companies' powerful lobbying arm, the Pharmaceutical Research and Manufacturers of America (PhRMA, pronounced "pharma") spends more than $150 million a year to fight attempts by the states and the federal governments to impose price restraints for prescription drugs. It's developing into a classic political battle between a powerful industry and unhappy constituents writing or calling their legislators for help.

Testifying before state legislatures and Congress, the drug companies continue to claim that they need to preserve their pricing schedules to provide money for research. But according to the Families USA study, the top nine pharmaceutical manufacturers spent more than twice as much on marketing, advertising, and administration as on research. That's where the big money goes, to advertising and marketing. You can't watch a half hour of television without seeing repeated pitches for the latest drug for relief of indigestion, allergies, and arthritis pain.

One state government after another appears to be rejecting the pharmaceutical industry's lobby line that higher consumer prices are needed to bolster research. Testimony by consumer groups and individuals is coming through loud and clear: Something has to be done to make more medicines readily available to modest-income constituents.

## Read It and Weep

"Profiting from Pain" is a riveting "by-the-numbers" report on who's making money off the poor, the sick, the elderly, and the chronically ill. It may not surprise you to learn that corporate profits and executive salaries in the pharmaceutical industry are sky-high, but the actual numbers may take your breath away.

While the industry claims that any price controls will deplete funds for necessary research and development, they're not telling you the truth. Before they ever need to trim their R&D budgets, these companies could easily reduce the billions they spend on marketing, advertising, and administration. Bristol Myers Squibb, for example, allots only 12 percent of its revenue to research, while it lavishes 27 percent on marketing and advertising. Some of the numbers are even more disturbing. Pharmacia spends 44 percent of its revenue on pushing its products but only 16 percent on the science and safety required to bring them to market. It's apparent that pharmaceutical companies spend so much money on TV commercials and promotions because they work. People do ask their doctors about Nexium, Clarinex, and other high-exposure products. You can't force the drug companies to cut down or cut out their advertising. And legislation to limit prescription drug advertising is not even being considered by Congress. With *Smart Medicine*, however, you can become an educated consumer, empowered to make your own drug choices that are based on gathering solid information and not on some smooth-talking pitch on television.

Perhaps the companies could also bring the prices of their products into line if they weren't paying their executives millions of dollars in salary and stock options. In 2001 average executive compensation, not including unexercised stock options, ranged from a high of $16 million at Pfizer to nearly $2 million for executives at Merck.

Want to read more? Go to www.familiesusa.org. Search for "profiting from pain" and you can download a file of the entire report. It's a good idea to know what you're dealing with.

## Average and Total Compensation for Highest-Paid Executives, Exclusive of Unexercised Stock Options

| Company | Average Compensation | Total Compensation for Highest-Paid Executives |
|---|---|---|
| Pfizer, Inc. | $15,688,335 | $94,130,007 |
| Bristol-Myers Squibb Co. | $14,874,834 | $89,249,005 |
| Wyeth | $9,144,196 | $54,865,177 |
| Allergan, Inc. | $4,536,450 | $27,218,697 |
| Abbott Laboratories | $4,247,409 | $21,237,047 |
| Schering-Plough Corp. | $3,724,997 | $22,349,981 |
| Pharmacia Corp. | $2,568,125 | $12,840,623 |
| Eli Lilly & Co. | $2,344,902 | $11,724,511 |
| Merck & Co., Inc. | $1,971,055 | $9,855,273 |
| **Total** | | **$343,470,321** |

From "Profiting from Pain: Where Prescription Drug Dollars Go,"
© 2002. Courtesy of Families USA and used by permission.

## WHO HAS THE PURCHASING POWER?

In partnership with the federal government, the states maintain and manage Medicaid health plans for low-income citizens. These medical plans, unlike Medicare, cover the total bill for prescription drug purchases. To be included in the various states' Medicaid contracts, the pharmaceutical companies have to provide serious discounts. The states get the best possible prices, and the companies get steady, long-term revenue.

But the bulk-purchasing power didn't stop there. Some enterprising members of Maine's legislature came up with a bill that would expand the state's already proven bulk-purchasing clout to include all of Maine's citizens who have modest incomes. It passed by a wide margin. Not surprisingly, the drug companies were shocked. Their association, PhRMA, challenged the Maine initiative in court and lost. The case went to the federal appeals court, and the companies still lost. They even took it all the way up to the United States Supreme Court—and lost again.

So citizens of Maine whose incomes are within 350 percent of the poverty level—$31,500 a year for singles and $42,000 a year for couples—can now get a significant break on prescriptions at their pharmacies. In general, the state's bulk-purchasing power knocked prices down by as much as 60 percent. So, if you were paying $100 for a prescribed medication for a heart condition, blood pressure, pain relief, indigestion, allergies, or whatever, you would now pay approximately $25.

Maine wasn't the only state to take action and fight prescription drug price inflation. Industry lawyers and lobbyists watched with alarm as a growing number of states began moving to follow Maine's lead. At least eighteen other state legislatures started writing laws to exert their government purchasing power to bring down drug costs for their constituents. It was the first time the pharmaceutical industry's lawyers and lobbyists suffered such a major setback. One jubilant Maine legislator, David LeMoine, who helped pass the bulk-purchasing discount law, said:

"They [the industry] spent tremendous amounts of money lobbying against our efforts to bring down drug costs. They took out newspaper ads, [ran] TV commercials, and sent legions of lobbyists out to collar members in the halls. But in Maine it backfired and our media exposed the powerful, out-of-state lobbyists as if they were aliens moving in on us."

Other New England states, plus New York and New Jersey, are working on a grand-scale, bulk-buyer consortium to get the best possible drug prices for their modest-income citizens. The Department of Veteran Affairs has long used its bulk-purchasing power to negotiate very substantial discounts from retail prices. (If you've ever served in the military and you haven't exercised this benefit, contact the nearest VA office to see if you qualify for this valuable drug assistance.)

## OREGON'S LIST OF LESS EXPENSIVE OPTIONS

The Oregon Health Resources Commission has gone in an entirely different direction to bring down prescription drug costs for its consumers. The Oregon plan

## For High Cholesterol (Statin) Drugs*

| Proprietary Drug Name (generic in bold) | Active Ingredient | Average price for 30-day supply** |
|---|---|---|
| Lescol | Fluvastatin | $63 |
| **Lovastatin** | Lovastatin | $69 |
| Lescol XL (controlled release) | Fluvastatin | $77 |
| Crestor | Rosuvastatin | $80 |
| Lipitor | Atorvastatin | $89 |
| Altocor (controlled release) | Lovastatin | $68 |
| Mevacor | Lovastatin | $98 |
| Pravachol | Pravastatin | $113 |
| Zocor | Simvastatin | $120 |

## For Muscle Spasm (Skeletal Muscle Relaxant) Drugs*

| Proprietary Drug Name (generic in bold) | Active Ingredient | Average price for 30-day supply** |
|---|---|---|
| **Chlorzoxazone** | Chlorzoxazone | $36 |
| **Baclofen** | Baclofen | $40 |
| Flexeril | Cyclobenzaprine | $70 |
| Norgesic | Orphenadrine with asprin and caffeine | $75 (low volume) |
| Dantrium | Dantrolene | $100 |
| Norflex | Orphenadrine | $105 (low volume) |
| Skelaxin | Metaxalone | $112 |
| Soma | Carisoprodol | $334 |

## For Joint/Muscle Pain—Arthritis (Non-Steroidal Anti-Inflammatory) Drugs*

| Proprietary Drug Name (generic in bold) | Active Ingredient | Average price for 30-day supply** |
|---|---|---|
| **Ibuprofen** | Ibruprofen | $19 |
| **Indomethacin** | Indomethacin | $26 |
| Motrin | Ibuprofen | $31 |
| **Naproxen** | Naproxen | $31 |
| **Naproxen Sodium** | Naproxen Sodium | $41 |
| **Diclofenac Sodium** | Diclofenac Sodium | $44 |
| Vioxx | Rofecoxib | $98 |
| Bextra | Valdecoxib | $102 |
| Celebrex | Celecoxib | $104 |
| Voltaren | Diclofenac Sodium | $117 |
| Cataflam | Diclofenac Potassium | $155 |

*Please note that these are not complete lists. For the complete AARP list of these classifications of drugs and for the other six classifications studies by the Oregon Health Resources Commission and the AARP, please visit the Web site at www.aarp.org/or/rx.

**Readers are cautioned that actual costs may be higher or lower based on the drug strength, dosing frequency, and other factors. Data was gathered from over 50,000 pharmacies nationwide from the period of 6/1/03 to 8/31/03.

Source for all formulary tables: Drugs identified through Oregon Health Resources Commission — Cost data through AARP Pharmacy Service from United Healthcare. Reprinted by permission.

provides a detailed comparison list (officially called a "formulary"). It lists names of drugs that have been laboratory proven to have the same therapeutic effect, but may be cheaper. For example, the Oregon formulary shows that a lesser-known acid indigestion medicine (Protonix, made by Wyeth) had the same effect as the widely advertised Nexium, made by AstraZenica, but cost only half as much. Lovastatin, a cholesterol control medicine, was rated a best buy over Mevacor and Pravachol. And for arthritis pain relief, a month's supply of generic ibuprofen costs only $19 as compared with the media-hyped Celebrex, which costs a whopping $104 for a month's supply.

Initially this information was aimed at Oregon physicians to guide them in prescribing the best medicine at the best price for their patients. The idea was to just click on a Web site and pick the top-rated drug (which was marked with stars). If physicians wanted a higher-priced drug, they had to specify why it was necessary.

Then the Oregon plan, in effect, went nationwide when AARP (formerly the American Association of Retired Persons) provided a link on its Web site in Oregon and eventually made the information available to its members around the country. Michigan now has a similar plan, and other states are looking into launching their own lists. Call your state senator or representative and find out if physicians and consumers in your state will soon have access to formulary, best-buy, prescription drug lists.

The AARP added prices to the drugs listed in the Oregon plan based on data gathered from 50,000 pharmacies nationwide. There may be a reason why you need a more expensive medicine, but you can save a lot of money by treating chronic pain with $27-a-month Methadose (Methadone), for instance, than with $266-a-month Duragesic patch (Fentanyl). According to the Oregon plan, Methadone and Fentanyl have been laboratory proven to have the same therapeutic effect. This list, then, lets you know what are the less-expensive drugs to treat your condition. You will need to check with your doctor to see if they are right for you.

## A GROWING POLITICAL UPROAR

You can imagine what PhRMA and the major drug manufacturers thought about giving consumers "inside" information involving comparable drugs and competitive pricing. They sent out legions of lobbyists to try to regain control of what some viewed as proprietary, professional knowledge.

"At the end of the legislature session, there was one pharmaceutical lobbyist for every three legislators," pointed out Kathleen M. Weaver, M.D., director of the Oregon plan. According to Dr. Weaver, they even tried to organize "citizen groups" to show grass roots opposition to the plan to imply that the lower-cost drugs were inferior. There were the write-in campaigns in which Oregon's formulary committee received more than 140 "form" letters from physicians claiming they had to have the more expensive drugs rather than the designated lower-cost products. The doctors went along with the pharmaceutical companies' campaigns because, according to Dr. Weaver, "they were told that the lower-cost products were inferior substitutions for the real thing which, of course, was false."

## THE CANADIAN CAPER

In Minnesota no such bulk-purchasing program or comparison list seemed necessary. Instead, some citizens discovered that they could cut their drug costs in half by filling their prescriptions at Canadian pharmacies just across the border. These pioneer "border-crossers" started a movement that began as a trickle and grew into a torrent as word spread.

It didn't seem to matter to anyone that purchasing prescription drugs across the border and driving back home with them was technically illegal. Americans are not supposed to bring large supplies of any prescription drugs into the United States from abroad. However, customs officials essentially "wink" at the practice because the returning citizens are buying the drugs for personal use and not for resale.

Not surprisingly, American drug manufacturers have sought to plug the Canadian leak in the profit-making dam because they see it as a clear threat to the bottom line. They became even more alarmed when Minnesotans found ways to get their prescriptions filled by Canadian pharmacies *without* spending the time and money to cross the border. Creative consumer groups worked with import-export lawyers to draft documents that permit prescription drug purchases to be mailed directly to the patient or to a medical office in the United States.

You can imagine the turmoil this caused among the drug manufacturers. According to Lee J. Craczyk, legislative director for the St. Paul-based Minnesota Senior Federation, "the drug companies threatened to cut back shipments to the Canadian distributors who were, in effect, exporting drug products they had originally imported from the United States."

The American companies whose products were involved in the Canadian import-export maneuver didn't give up easily. They increased the prices of drug products that were being shipped to Canada and then added a new wrinkle: The drug companies tried to prevent Americans from buying drugs in Canada by requiring them to have special coupons which were available only to Canadian citizens. It became too convoluted, though, and quickly fizzled. The rules seem to keep changing from day to day. Other reimportation schemes are in the works, as are efforts to arrange bulk purchasing by states and towns across the United States.

On November 7, 2003, U.S. District Court Judge Claire Eagan tried to cut off one kind of importation method. The judge shut down RxDepot, a company operating storefront emporiums in Oklahoma that took prescription orders and faxed them to Canada. The orders were filled in Canada at deep discounts and shipped back to the store. Judge Eagan wrote, "This court is not unsympathetic to the predicament faced by individuals who cannot afford their prescription drugs at U.S. prices. However, the defendants are able to offer lower prices only because they facilitate illegal activity determined by Congress to harm the public interest." She cited RxDepot for "openly and notoriously" violating the law, but Carl Moore, founder of the Tulsa-based chain, announced he would appeal the decision. "There's a drug crisis in this country due to the pricing and price gouging that goes on. I'm going to do my part to see drug prices lowered in this country," Moore said. Since the stores were not licensed for regular commerce, he will probably lose the appeal.

A few other similar companies are still operating. And even if they are shut down for not following commerce regulations, others will find a way to work within the rules. This may sound as though the ability to get your prescriptions filled over the border is about to end. By mail, that may be the case, but right now you can still bring in a three-month's supply for personal use.

This matter is still up in the air. As of this publication it is still legal to purchase drugs from Canada and Mexico, but that could all change. To stay up to date with this pricing war, join a consumer watchdog group such as AARP, Families USA, the Committee to Preserve Social Security and Medicare, the National Council on the Aging, or other organizations listed in the Appendix.

## SELECTING GENERIC DRUGS

The political battle about dispensing generic drugs continues between the pharmaceutical manufacturers and state governments, but the initial skirmishes in this war started three decades ago. The American Pharmacists Association (formerly the American Pharmaceutical Association) tried for years to get legislation passed that would let a qualified pharmacist dispense the generic equivalent of a more costly brand name product to save the customer money. Naturally, the drug companies that created the brand name drugs did not want this to happen.

The drug manufacturers' lobbyists tried to convince lawmakers and the public that the companies that produced lower-cost, generic drugs were fly-by-night establishments. The "brand name" group created the impression that the people who were manufacturing and distributing the lower-cost drugs were using substandard production methods that put patients at risk. The same drug companies that were doing the finger pointing, however, were also making these supposedly poor-quality products. In some cases, they even owned the generic production companies about which they were publicly complaining. They wanted control of the high-scale market *and* the low-scale market for essentially the same product.

For now, it's up to consumers to request generics from physicians and to actively solicit the opinions of trusted pharmacists to find out if a generic equivalent is available to them.

## THE PATENT MONOPOLY TWIST

In chapter 3, you'll learn how a brand name drug comes to market and why manufacturers get a pricing monopoly on their brand name products that lasts the lifetime of their patents (seventeen years). Essentially, they are entitled to exclusivity for this period to earn back the costs of "innovation," the years of scientific effort to develop the product. It's similar (although shorter) to the copyright on books, for instance.

But the U.S. government allows a patent or a copyright to expire for the common good, so that a product or a literary work can be made widely available to its citizens for a lower cost. That's why you can buy a cheap paperback copy of a Dickens novel but you still have to pay full retail prices for a thriller by John Grisham.

Once a drug loses its initial patent, any company can manufacture it as a generic product at a lower cost to the consumer. But some pharmaceutical firms tweak or adjust the formula for the drug that's going off patent so it becomes a "new" brand name product—which then qualifies for another patent and seventeen more years of exclusivity.

Independent tests have shown that the "old" generic drug and the "new" brand name product provide virtually the same therapeutic effect. You just pay more for the brand name. This subterfuge was successful for quite a while, and still is in some cases, but some states have begun taking manufacturers to court and asking for millions of dollars in compensation for consumers who had to pay top dollar for drugs that could have been purchased for less.

Thirty-four states joined forces to sue several manufacturers, alleging that they manipulated the federal patent process to extend their monopolies on widely pre-scribed drugs by slightly adjusting the products' contents to receive new patents. In a negotiated settlement covering BuSpar, a widely prescribed anti-anxiety drug made by Bristol-Myers Squibb, the states were awarded $100 million to reimburse local Medicaid programs and individual consumers for having paid too high a price for their medicines.

"There's no question that consumers were denied the opportunity to pur-chase less expensive drugs," said Pennsylvania Attorney General Mike Fisher. In a similar case, Fisher said, Bristol Myers Squibb had to pay back $55 million in alleged overcharges for the cancer drug Taxol, when a generic equivalent cost considerably less money.

In another action, forty-nine states and the District of Columbia got a judgment requiring GlaxoSmithKline and the Bayer Corporation to pay a $329 million rebate to the regional governments' Medicaid programs and to consumers. New York got an $80 million settlement from Avantis Pharmaceuticals and the Andryx Corporation by successfully proving that the companies conspired to keep a less costly generic version of the blood pressure medication Cardizem CD off the market.

## THE FEDERAL THREAT

While the drug companies appear to be losing ground at the state government level, they are working hard and doing better in Washington. When Congress came up with legislation to provide a modest prescription drug benefit for Medicare patients, the drug companies lobbied to spread out the benefit management among private medical insurers so the government would have little or no leverage to negotiate bet-ter prices. The drug industry feared the federal government would use its potential bulk-purchasing power to extract significant price cuts. The companies wanted to avoid what happened in Maine, where the major discounts given to the Medicaid program were extended to include many other citizens who were not otherwise covered by medical insurance.

The benefit from the new legislation offers only modest help for individual citizens, but it will cost the government billions of dollars over time. Bulk-buying discounts could save the country some of those billions. Perhaps in the future the federal government may rewrite the regulations permitting it to exercise bulk-buying power, as did Maine and other state governments.

The annual struggle to balance the nation's budget means a constant search for new strategies to save more and spend less. Will taxes be raised to cover the red ink? Not likely. Instead the members of Congress may join those prescient states that took on the Goliaths and won.

## BENEFITS BAG

Benefits will be in play starting January 2006. Meanwhile, you can buy a prescription drug discount card that will provide savings of 15 percent or so off retail prices. Beneficiaries with incomes below $12,123 ($16,362 for couples) would also get $600 a year to help pay for prescription drugs in 2004 and 2005.

Beginning in 2006 private companies will administer drug benefits on a regional basis. There are two ways beneficiaries will be able to get their benefits. They will get new, separate policies for drugs or be able to use private health plans that also provide all their other medical needs.

The new Medicare prescription drug "policies" will work a lot like any other medical insurance. There will be a monthly premium of $35 and an annual deductible of $250. There will be somewhat confusing limits on how much benefits will cover. For spending up to $2,250 in total prescription costs, Medicare will pick up 75 percent of the tab.

There will be no coverage, however, for drug expenditures between $2,250 and $3,600. Why this interim group gets nothing is perplexing and, hopefully, might be rewritten before 2006. Having no reimbursement for certain expenditures might encourage patients to spend more on the higher cost brand names instead of their inexpensive generic counterpart. By spending more the patient can get over the $3,600 amount and receive 95 percent reimbursement.

There will be special help for those seniors whose income is just above the point where they would qualify for Medicaid, which would pay 100 percent for all their prescription drugs. Here's how it works. Individuals whose income is less than $12,123 a year (couples $16,362) and have less than $6,000 in assets would not have to pay the premiums and deductibles. They would pay only three dollars for each brand name drug and one dollar for each generic. And as a bonus, these lower income folks would be able to avoid that nasty gap in annual expenditures between $2,250 and $3,600 where you don't get any reimbursement.

The prescription drug benefits can be confusing and may require help from someone who has studied the rules and regulations. You can contact your physician or your area agency on aging (found under county or city government listing in your phone book).

## ARE BETTER BENEFITS ON THE WAY?

Is this move by Congress to provide prescription drug benefits for Medicare beneficiaries a one-shot deal or is it just the beginning of some Medicare tune-ups in upcoming years? There's no question that these new benefits have whetted the appetites of seniors and politicians alike. Some say this is a good start but more needs to be done. Senator John Edwards (D-NC), among others in Congress, would like to see these items in future Medicare legislation:

- Disclosure requirements for direct-to-consumer prescription drug commercials and print ads where pharmaceutical companies would have to include the effectiveness of any given medication compared with similar products on the market.

- Increased negotiations between federal and state governments and the pharmaceutical companies to bargain for reduced prices for Medicare beneficiaries.

- A review of prescription drug patent laws that could provide consumers with earlier access to lower-cost generic medicines.

## How Did We Get Here from There?

If we do not learn from history, we are condemned to repeat it, the saying goes. But does the history of the pharmaceutical industry hold the solution to our range of prescription drug political concerns?

We've come a long way from the basement chemical laboratories with their vials, test tubes, and gas burners, and the business of discovering and distributing drugs has grown ever more complex. There's a cornucopia of medicines out there behind the pharmacy counter and along drugstore aisles. There's much more to discover about those drugs—how they are developed, marketed, and sold through a variety of different channels. It's important to learn all you can about getting the right drug for the best price. In the next section of *Smart Medicine* you'll find out all about brand name drugs, generic drugs, over-the-counter products, and the plethora of herbal remedies, vitamins, and minerals—and you'll learn what it takes to keep yourself safe.

# UNDERSTANDING DRUGS

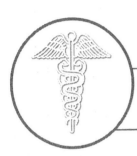

## THREE

## BRAND NAME DRUGS

We know that the history of the American pharmaceutical industry goes back to our earliest days as a nation. The business of selling medicines evolved into one where an emphasis on research was necessary to ensure growth and profits over time. As scientists began to understand more about biology and developed instruments that provided ever more intricate insights into the microscopic villains that cause disease in the human body, the art and craft of making medicines advanced rapidly.

But how are these new drugs discovered? Where and how are these "miracles" born? "We're on the cutting edge of the biological sciences," explained Rhoda Gruen, Ph.D., who works in research and development at pharmaceutical firm Hoffmann-LaRoche, Inc., in a 1999 FDA report: "We suck up new information like a sponge. Everything we do is subject to change as new scientific information becomes known."

Research is complex, costly, and time-consuming, and success is never a given. Thousands of different chemical combinations must be manufactured and tested over and over to find the "needle in the haystack," the one version that may have the power to save lives. The FDA estimates that it takes an average of eight and a half years to study and test a new drug before it can receive agency approval to be sold to the public. A 1993 report by the Congressional Office of Technology Assessment said that companies spend more than $350 million to develop a new drug, and it's more than likely that those costs have escalated since then. Hoffmann-LaRoche, for example, spends about a billion dollars annually on worldwide research into new products.

How does it all begin? Each drug follows a different journey. Scientists begin asking questions about body functions and the steps of the disease process. By charting these "events" along a timeline, they hope to understand what causes each step and what might halt that development. They try to break down what is happening at the cellular and molecular levels, then target that particular moment in the course of the disease—and make their stand.

*From Test Tube to Patient*, a lengthy report from the Center for Drug Evaluation and Research, describes how this works by zeroing in on cholesterol. This waxy substance occurs naturally in the body, but too much of it can build up on the inner walls of blood vessels, clogging the arteries that send blood to the heart, and at its worst, preventing the flow of oxygen and nutrients. The result is a heart attack.

Most of the drugs that tried to tackle this particular problem had nasty side effects or were simply too toxic in the amounts required. Others just didn't get to the "heart" of the problem in time. What was needed was a drug that would tackle cholesterol buildup much earlier in the timeline.

Scientists at many different companies worked for years to understand how and why the body produces cholesterol and if it has any use. They discovered "more than twenty biochemical reactions necessary for the body to make cholesterol, along with the enzymes required at each step to turn one chemical into the next one in the chain," explained Eve Slater, M.D., former executive vice president for worldwide regulatory affairs for Merck. "The challenge," she continued, "was to find a point at which a drug could effectively lower cholesterol production early enough to make a difference."

By the 1970s scientists had isolated an early link in the cholesterol "chain," a chemical called mevalonic acid and an enzyme called HMG-CoA, which produced this chemical. They needed a drug that would inhibit HMG-CoA from doing its job or prevent cells from properly reacting to the enzyme.

The advent of computers made testing easier in some ways, allowing simulations of how different compounds worked so researchers could try to design chemicals to prevent them from working that way. These high-tech changes made some of the work go faster, but the process was still extraordinarily lengthy.

This story, one among many told in the report, describes the discovery of a fungus that could prevent the enzyme from working. Not until the 1980s and 1990s did the cholesterol-fighting drugs Mevacor and Zocor arrive on the market, but they were among the most profitable drugs ever developed by Merck.

Not every such odyssey has a happy ending. Many drugs are set aside and research stopped because tests show that the compound is unsafe, doesn't work, or isn't well absorbed by the body. Yet some drugs that are shelved for years because they don't work on a particular disease may be reclaimed, researched further, and discovered to work on an unrelated condition.

## DIARY OF A DRUG

The journey of a drug from discovery to your medicine cabinet is complex: It takes a long time and costs a tremendous amount of money. That's the primary reason the drug belongs exclusively to its "innovator company" for years before it can be made available in generic form.

Novartis Pharmaceuticals originally discovered Gleevec (imatinib mesylate)—a drug used to treat Philadelphia chromosome positive (Ph+) chronic myeloid leukemia (CML)—in 1992. It then took nine years before the FDA approved the drug. When they announced approval of the drug, based on "three separate studies in about 1,000 patients," the FDA press release sought to explain the government's accelerated approval of this new cancer protocol. "FDA and Novartis, the drug's manufacturer, should be commended for the rapid development and review that will make this product available soon for the leukemia patients who desperately need it," said Health and Human Services Secretary Tommy G. Thompson.

The FDA approved Gleevec under its "orphan" drug program, which provides financial incentives to pharmaceutical companies to develop drugs to treat such rare diseases as CML. In this case it approved the drugs based on clinical trials that showed Gleevec "to reduce substantially the level of cancerous cells in the bone marrow and blood of treated patients."

Some in the media referred to Gleevec as a "magic bullet" because it was believed to target only the enzymes in the body that allow cancerous cells to grow, not a patient's normal healthy cells.

The FDA's acting deputy principal commissioner at the time, Bernard A. Schwetz,

D.V.M., was frank in noting the research still to come. "Although the long-term benefits of the drug are not yet known, early studies have shown that Gleevec will offer a significant improvement for many patients," he stated in the press release. "However," he added, "further studies are needed to evaluate whether Gleevec provides an actual clinical benefit, such as improved survival, as well as to examine its effect when used in early stage disease."

Like many major pharmaceutical companies, Novartis provides a Web site (www.gleevec.com) with information on the drug for both patients and health- care professionals. The site explains who should take this drug and how it works.

FDA approval in 2001 was only the first step for this cancer drug. In February 2002 Gleevec was granted accelerated approval for treating gastrointestinal stromal cancer. Then in May 2003, the FDA announced that Gleevec had been approved for treating pediatric patients with the Philadelphia chromosome positive (Ph+) chronic myeloid leukemia, which affects about 2 percent of all children diagnosed with leukemia. The

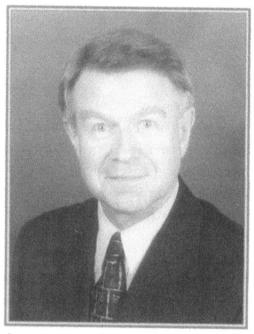

*Bernard A. Schwetz, D.V.M.*
Photo courtesy of the Food & Drug Administration

FDA press release noted that Gleevec was "indicated for children whose disease has recurred after stem cell transplant or who are resistant to interferon alpha therapy."

FDA Commissioner Mark B. McClellan, M.D., Ph.D., explained why a drug might receive a speedier-than-typical approval by the FDA. "Gleevec was originally granted accelerated approval two years ago for certain kinds of leukemia in adults, and now has been shown to be a valuable treatment for certain leukemias in children that do not respond to other treatments. With follow-up studies to confirm its benefits, Gleevec illustrates the type of significant medical advance for children that can be achieved quickly under FDA's accelerated approval program."

## The Gleevec Story

Drugs are created under many different circumstances. Some drugs are born as the result of a happy accident in a laboratory or a chance discovery in the field. But most require decades of scientific research by many people whose combined efforts may ultimately lead to a "miracle" medicine that treats a serious disease, which is how some reports described the cancer drug Gleevec.

In the case of Gleevec, the story really begins around 1960, when researchers studying the blood of chronic myeloid leukemia patients observed abnormalities on chromosome 22, which was named the Philadelphia chromosome. During the next thirty years, scientists continued to study the chromosome and ultimately found that a gene that produces a mutated protein caused this type of leukemia in laboratory mice. Here's how the process goes.

1. **Drug discovery.** In 1992 the drug was first made in Novartis Laboratories, and laboratory studies began in 1993. At that point the investigatory drug was called STI571.

2. **Initial testing.** Five years later, in 1998, and after initial efforts to develop the drug, laboratory tests showed that a small group of patients who had failed to improve after interferon-alpha therapy (all that was available at the time to treat this form of the disease) responded to Gleevec.

3. **Expanded testing.** From 1999 to 2000 researchers gathered data from a larger group of patients at the University of Maryland, University of Minnesota, and University of Texas Southwestern Medical Center. This work confirmed earlier findings and showed that patients improved significantly when treated with Gleevec.

4. **Initial approval.** In May 2001 the FDA approved Gleevec for patients who failed to improve after interferon therapy.

5. **Extended approval.** By the fall of 2001, the European Union and Japan approved Gleevec.

6. **FDA final approval.** By the end of 2001, the drug was approved for all patients suffering from inoperable and metastatic (widespread) chronic myeloid leukemia .

Dr. McClellan added that this was the first approval of a new pediatric cancer drug in more than ten years. The FDA also noted that, as a condition of approval, Novartis had agreed to conduct pediatric studies after approval to gain greater insight into the drug's use in children.

The FDA put Gleevec on a fast track because it offered the promise of a new treatment for a disease not responding to available medications. Federal regulations allow the FDA to speed up the approval of some drugs for life-threatening illnesses when the new drug appears to be a significant improvement over products currently on the market.

Other drugs may wait years longer for approval. Fast track or slow track, bringing drugs from initial testing to the marketplace costs tens of millions of dollars. Exact figures spent for Gleevec research and development are guarded by the manufacturer, but considering the years invested in its

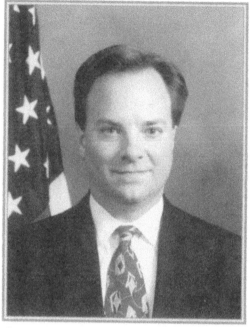

Commissioner Mark B. McClellan, M.D., Ph.D.
Photo courtesy of the Food & Drug Administration

development, the hundreds of scientists and technicians involved in its study, and the costs of building plants to manufacture the chemical ingredients (not to mention the raw materials required), it's easy to see that creating, testing, and marketing a brand-new brand name drug is expensive.

## WHO PAYS TO DEVELOP A DRUG?

The money for research comes from more than one source. In the case of Gleevec, the financing for the earliest scientific studies likely came from the government (through National Institutes of Health grants), from foundations whose missions included support for scientific research into drugs to treat cancer, even from individuals and institutions with a stake in the outcome.

Think about it for a moment. Have you ever participated in your local Race for the Cure? The money raised by entry fees and donations goes to the Susan G. Komen Foundation, which funnels it to research and education programs around the country. While that foundation's focus is on breast cancer, other groups raise funds for all kinds of cancers (American Cancer Society, for instance). Much of the money spent on research, however, comes from the pharmaceutical company's own resources—their way of investing in the future. New and better medications are the key to company growth and increased profits.

If you're interested in learning more about the intricate route traveled by each newly developed drug, you can order or download a 100-page brochure called *From Test Tube to Patient: Improving Health through Human Drugs* from the FDA Web site (www.FDA.gov). This 1999 report explains how the Center for Drug Evaluation and Research within this important government agency operates on your behalf. Topics covered in its pages include:

- Why Should the FDA Regulate Drugs?
- The Beginnings: Laboratory and Animal Studies
- Testing Drugs on People
- How CDER Approves New Drugs
- Getting Outside Advice for Close Calls
- How the FDA Ensures Equivalence of Generic Drugs
- When a Drug Is in Short Supply
- TV Drug Ads That Make Sense
- Pediatric Drug Studies: Protecting Pint-Sized Patients
- Medications and Older Adults
- A Dose of Clear Directions for Prescription Drug Users
- New Drug Labels Spell It Out Simply

The brochure also has chapters on how the FDA operates; how Medwatch, the FDA's Medical Product Safety program, works; and more about how this consumer watchdog agency is committed to bringing the public safe and effective drugs. It provides important insights about how the FDA continually revises its methods. For instance, beginning in 1994, the agency implemented new requirements that women and minorities be adequately represented in research studies, because drugs may work differently for patients who are not white or male. The symptoms of a heart attack are often different for female patients, who may be sent home from the emergency room after complaining of "nonstandard" chest pain when in fact they are experiencing a coronary event. Before increased women's inclusion in medical studies, many women succumbed to heart attacks because their symptoms were different from those men experienced. By including women in the studies, doctors became familiar with the signs that indicate when a woman is having a heart attack. Now doctors perform more tests when women complain of nonstandard chest pain.

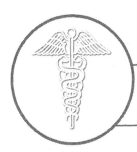

## FOUR

## GENERIC DRUGS

When a pharmaceutical company researches and tests a new drug and goes through the procedures to earn FDA approval for that drug, the company earns the right to patent, name, and protect its discovery—but that trademark protection doesn't last forever.

After seventeen years, as mentioned earlier, the company loses exclusivity, and other companies are permitted to produce the drug. (But first they have to prove they can correctly and safely manufacture the drug's specific chemical composition, and that's not always easy.) This is why consumers can purchase different versions of medications such as ibuprofen or acetaminophen. A pharmacy, for example, may decide to sell its own brand of the drug at a lower price than a well-known brand such as Advil (ibuprofen) or Tylenol (acetaminophen).

But many consumers wonder whether they're buying a watered-down version of the "real thing" when they purchase 250 extra-strength acetaminophen caplets with the Eckerd name on them for only $12.79, instead of the smaller, 150-caplet bottle of Tylenol sitting right next to it that costs $11.99. One hundred more pills for less than a dollar more? It's easy to feel suspicious, but you don't have to.

According to the FDA when a new drug is developed, it has two names—the chemical or generic name and the trademarked brand name that is used to market the drug. The company that develops the drug owns the rights to it—for a period of time. (In most cases, it is seventeen years, but sometimes a drug has several different patents and may be protected for a longer period.) When the patent has run out, other companies are permitted to develop and sell their own versions of the chemical compound.

A generic drug, which could be available only by prescription or in an over-the-counter (OTC) version, usually costs less than its brand name cousin because of marketing competition among the manufacturers. But it is required to contain exactly the same active ingredients. It has to be just as potent as the original medication, and even if it looks very different from the original drug, it has to work in the same way as the brand name drug.

In fact no company is allowed to sell a generic drug until it proves to the FDA that its medication contains the same ingredients in the same size dose as the original, and that it performs exactly the same way in the body as the brand name product. Approval for generic drugs requires a rigorous, multistep process that includes reviewing research and approving the plant where the drug will be manufactured. The manufacturers of generic drugs don't have to reproduce the original clinical trials that the company that created the drug did, but the product must be chemically identical—what the FDA calls "bioequivalent."

The FDA monitors both brand name and generic drugs, and inspectors require generics to demonstrate the same quality and consistency as the brand name medications. They also insist that the generic drugs meet the same standards of safety.

Generic drugs frequently look different than the original, brand name products, including shape, size, color, even flavor, but they do not affect the way the drug is metabolized by the body. The things that affect color or flavor, for example, are "inactive" ingredients.

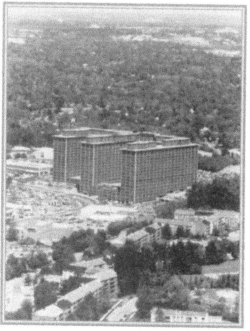

The FDA's Parklawn Building in which research is done
Photo courtesy of the Food & Drug Administration

## FDA Requirements for Generic Drugs

According to an FDA Center for Drug Evaluation and Research (CDER) bulletin, drug products must meet eight basic requirements before they can be officially designated as generic. To check out FDA and CDER bulletins, go to the agency's Web site (www.fda.gov).

- Generic drugs must have the same active ingredients and the same strength as the brand name product.

- Generic drugs must have the same dosage form (for example, tablets, liquids) and must be administered in the same way.

- Generic drug manufacturers must show that a generic drug is bioequivalent to the brand name drug—delivering the same amount of active ingredients into a patient's bloodstream in the same amount of time.

- Generic drug labeling must be essentially the same as the labeling of the brand name drug, although listing the drug's chemical name, not the brand.

- Generic drug manufacturers must fully document the generic drug's chemistry, manufacturing steps, and quality control measures.

- Firms must assure the FDA that the raw materials and finished product meet specifications of the U.S. Pharmacopoeia, the organization that sets standards for drug purity in the United States.

- Firms must show that a generic drug will remain potent and unchanged until the expiration date on the label.

- Firms must comply with federal regulations for good manufacturing practices and provide the FDA a full description of facilities they use to manufacture, process, test, package, and label the drug. The FDA inspects manufacturing facilities to ensure compliance.

Interestingly, about half of all generic drugs are produced by the same companies that developed the brand-new drugs in the first place. Also some drugs are never released in generic versions because their production is too complex or expensive.

## WHY ARE GENERIC DRUGS SO MUCH LESS EXPENSIVE?

Among the reasons for the lower prices of generic drugs is that you are no longer paying for two significant costs: the pharmaceutical company's extensive research to develop the original drug and the enormous advertising budgets required to make physicians and consumers intimately aware of the product. Another important reason for lowered costs is competition. When more than one company is competing for customers, they tend to lower the price as an incentive to buy their product.

When patent protection expires and companies start producing generic versions of the drug, those companies, which are only manufacturing that product, have modest research costs and lower marketing budgets, because they focus their promotional efforts on informing physicians and pharmacists that a generic version is available. As the consumer, you're paying simply for the product you're buying and not for the costly advertising.

For example, Pfizer makes and sells Lipitor, whose chemical or generic name is atorvastatin calcium. For the length of its patent, Pfizer is the only company permitted to sell this cholesterol-lowering drug. Once that protection expires, other companies will be allowed to produce generic versions of the drug under the name atorvastatin calcium. It's quite a mouthful, but someday it may be as familiar to the general public as acetaminophen or ibuprofen.

## WHO MAKES GENERIC DRUGS?

The average consumer may be unaware of any companies whose primary business is making generic drugs, as their public profiles tend to be much lower. But as many of them are public companies, it's possible to learn quite a lot by studying their corporate Web sites or other sources of investment information.

For example, Jeff Fischer of *The Motley Fool* investment advice Web site (www.fool.com) profiled Mylan Labs in spring 2003. Selecting it for its strong position in the generic drug industry, he described Mylan as a forty-year-old company that made both brand name and generic drugs. Mylan manufactures more than 100 different generic drugs in more than 250 different dosage strengths. It also distributes for other companies in addition to developing and marketing its own products. Its two dozen brand name products include Phenytek for seizure control, Mentax (an antifungal cream), and Amnesteem for severe acne; its generics include albuterol, the widely used asthma medication, and many others, producing generic-only sales of more than $750 million in a nine-month period.

## THE LEGISLATION
## THAT MAKES GENERIC DRUGS VIABLE

In 1984 Congress passed the Hatch-Waxman Act, also known as the Drug Price Competition and Patent Term Restoration Act of 1984. The Act said that generic drug companies don't have to repeat expensive clinical trials, a tremendous savings in time and expense. In the September-October issue of the *FDA Consumer* magazine, Gary Buehler, R.Ph., director of the FDA's Office of Generic Drugs, said, "The Hatch-Waxman Act essentially created the generic drug industry." Twenty years ago, only 12 percent of all prescriptions were for generic drugs. Now, generics represent almost 51 percent of all prescriptions in the United States, according to the Generic Pharmaceutical Association.

"The law paved the way for many more generic drugs because, rather than repeating research, generic drug companies instead must show the FDA that their drugs are bioequivalent to the brand name drug," Buehler said. Bioequivalent drugs are drugs with essentially the same bioavailability—quantity of active ingredient and rate of absorption or activation.

What does that mean? Scientists measure how a generic drug does the job, checking the amount of the generic drug in the bloodstream and how long it takes to get there. Then they compare that measurement to how the brand name drug works. "Innovator" companies, what the FDA calls the firms that actually develop and research new drugs, are required to submit more comprehensive applications, while generic companies submit abbreviated new drug applications. After showing that a generic drug has the same bioavailability as the brand name drug, generic companies also must demonstrate that their products have the same active ingredient, follow the same quality manufacturing standards, and have similar labeling.

Buehler noted that the intense competition in the generic market not only keeps costs lower but actually encourages the efforts from the innovator companies to

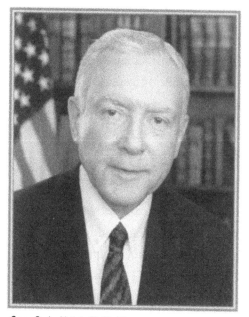

*Sen. Orrin Hatch (R-Utah)*
Photo courtesy of Senator Hatch's office

launch new drugs. "The law aims to protect the intellectual property rights of the innovator companies while at the same time encouraging the development of generic drugs," he said. It does this by allowing the FDA to grant a period of exclusivity to the first "generic challenger" of a brand name drug patent. The period of exclusivity is a period of time in which no other company can compete. This is done to encourage companies to come up with generic drugs to get the competition rolling.

The FDA has intensified its efforts to make generic drugs more accessible for all Americans. In June 2003 the FDA and Health and Human Services Secretary Tommy G. Thompson announced new FDA regulations aimed at streamlining the process of getting generic drugs to the public. The move is expected to save consumers $35 billion over the next decade, as well as lower costs for state Medicaid programs and employer insurance plans.

In addition the FDA launched an initiative called "Improving Access to Generic Drugs," which includes revamping the FDA's review process to make generic drugs available to consumers more quickly. President Bush's fiscal year 2004 budget request increased funding for the FDA's generic drug program by $13 million, the largest ever for that purpose—one-third more than the program's $45 million budget. The additional funds were expected to help speed generic drug reviews.

The FDA's revised rule, which went into effect in August 2003, is designed to close legal loopholes in the Hatch-Waxman Act that delay generic drug approval. For example, the new regulation allows only one thirty-month "stay" if an innovator company sues a generic company over patent issues. The FDA cannot approve the generic drug during such a stay. Unless the innovator sues within forty-five days of such notice, there is no thirty-month stay. Sometimes

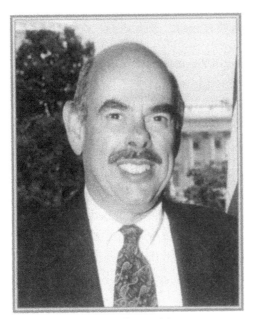

*Rep. Henry Waxman (D-California)*
Photo courtesy of Representative Waxman's office

pharmaceutical manufacturers keep getting thirty-month stays as long as possible. It's a delaying tactic that also gives them an excuse to launch the drug with the higher price tag.

The Federal Trade Commission (FTC) agreed with the FDA's new stance, noting that between 1994 and 2000 repeated stays delayed public access to several generic drugs. President Bush commented: "Our message to brand name manufacturers is clear: You deserve the fair rewards of your research and development; you do not have the right to keep generic drugs off the market for frivolous reasons." Other aspects of the new ruling aim to allow only patent applications related to active ingredients, approved uses of a drug, and the chemical formulations and compositions of a drug. Patents for packaging claims, for instance, may no longer be submitted during this process.

Some members of Congress wanted to close the loopholes that allowed for the continuous stays that in turn kept generic drugs from being approved. Bruce N. Kuhlik, PhRMA's senior vice president and general counsel, however, is in favor of keeping the current law as it is. When he testified before the Senate Judiciary Committee on June 17, 2003, he strongly advised against changes that might "undermine incentives for continued pharmaceutical innovation." Kuhlik expressed the belief that the Hatch-Waxman Act was already accomplishing its purpose of easing the launch of generic drugs into the marketplace.

Kuhlik claims the law provides incentives for companies to develop new drugs by allowing them to keep out competition. It has been the pharmaceutical industry's political standard that manufacturers need more money so they can spend more on research to develop new drugs. (See the Families USA chart on page 14.)

## New Generic Drugs Arrive Each Year

The FDA approved 321 new generic drugs in 2002—more than in any of the previous seven years, when approvals ranged from a low of 186 in 1999 to a high of 273 in 1997. With the class of 2002 included, statistics show it takes an average of twenty months for generic drug approvals. The goal is to shorten that time by several months by improving communication between the FDA and the applicant companies, so that minor problems and questions don't force lengthy delays in approval.

FDA Commissioner Mark B. McClellan, M.D., Ph.D., announced he will hire forty new staffers in order to get approval guidelines out to manufacturers faster and to help them submit proper applications the first time around instead of delaying the approval by having them redo the applications or by opening the door for lawsuits.

The FDA is also interested in building consumer confidence in generic drugs, and its consumer education ad campaign has featured bus advertising in Los Angeles, Chicago, and New York, as well as brochures and posters in pharmacies nationwide. The theme is "Generic Drugs: Safe. Effective. FDA Approved."

## Who Wants You to Buy Generic Drugs?

Until recently many consumers believed that insurers were primarily interested in saving money for the company, not their members, when they encouraged pharmacists and physicians to prescribe generic drugs. But as the cost of brand name drugs continued to rise, consumers joined the crusade and began asking for generics. When Blue Cross Blue Shield of Michigan launched a contest in 2001 to educate consumers about the quality and value of generic drugs, it agreed to feature the pharmacies and pharmacists who increased their rate of dispensing generic drugs the most in a $1 million ad campaign. Savings to state residents were estimated at $25 million to $30 million in that year alone. The campaign featured the slogan, "Generic Drugs—The Unadvertised Brand."

If the goal is making health care more affordable for Americans, making generic drugs available easily and reliably is key to reducing medical costs. A 2002 study by the Schneider Institute for Health Policy at Brandeis University determined that if Medicare increased its rate of generic drug use to that of many private health-care plans, its 40 million clients might save more than $14 billion in just one year.

"Substantial savings can be realized if generic drug incentive techniques used in the private sector are broadly applied within a Medicare prescription drug program," said Stanley Wallack, human services research professor and director of The Schneider Institute for Health Policy at The Heller School for Social Policy and Management, in a press release. Over a ten-year period, that could result in $250 billion savings of the estimated $1.5 trillion costs of prescription drugs.

Anthem Prescription Management, the Blue Cross and Blue Shield licensee for nine states, manages pharmacy benefits for millions of health-care plan members. In 2003 it launched a generics "sampling" program in New Hampshire called "Think Generics," and then extended the program to Anthem members in Colorado, Indiana, Kentucky, Maine, Nevada, and Ohio.

With Think Generics, doctors in the network are given "sample request" cards to offer their patients. Using the cards, members may receive free samples of different generic medicines at their local pharmacies. Health plan members receive a complimentary supply of their first prescription order for the prescribed generic medication, and the pharmacy is reimbursed by sending a claim to Anthem. The drugs on the sampling list include generic versions of many of the most commonly prescribed medications, offering tremendous potential savings to both members and their health plans. "Appropriate use of generics represents one of the most significant savings opportunities for our health plan members," said Sam Nussbaum, M.D., Anthem's chief medical officer. "Think Generics is designed to encourage a dialogue between physicians and their patients about the potential advantages of using generic prescription medications rather than the more expensive brand alternatives."

The price differences between brand name drugs and generics are significant. According to a 2003 AARP study, for example, the brand name cholesterol-reducing drug Zocor, for a thirty-day supply, runs about $120. You can get a month's supply of the generic Lovastatin for around only $69. That's almost a 50 percent savings. The savings greatly increase if your ailment allows you to use an over-the-counter drug. In the New Hampshire "Think Generics" test, for a typical NSAID (nonsteroidal anti-inflammatory drug) the brand name prescription averaged $71.57 while the average cost of an over-the-counter NSAID was $7.82. That should be enough to motivate you to ask your pharmacist and physician what other drugs may be available.

## WHY DIDN'T I GET A GENERIC DRUG?

There are several possible reasons you were not offered a generic drug. First, your physician may not have known that a generic drug was available. Not all generics arrive on the market with fanfare, and doctors are extremely busy trying to see patients and keep up with current research in their fields. If you're handed a prescription with a drug name in capital letters, you're getting a brand name prescription drug. Take a moment before you leave the doctor's office to ask if a generic is available. If your doctor isn't certain, ask if the prescription can reflect that a generic may be used to fill this prescription if one is available.

The second reason is that unless your physician writes on your prescription that it may be filled with a generic drug, your pharmacist has no authority to do so. However, say you go to the drugstore to drop off your prescription. You take the time to ask the pharmacist if a generic is available. If the pharmacist says yes, hand over your physician's phone number and ask if the pharmacy can call the doctor to get permission to dispense the generic instead. Most pharmacies will agree to do so at your request.

Another reason not to prescribe or dispense a generic version of your prescription drug, suggests DrugDigest (www.drugdigest.org), one of the more comprehensive drug information Web sites, is allergies. If you have an allergy to something such as wheat, for example, you should not use a generic that happens to contain wheat fiber. (While a generic drug contains exactly the same active ingredients as the brand name drug, the inactive ingredients can differ.) If you know you have allergies, ask your pharmacist about what may be in your medication. Make sure it's noted on your medical chart at your doctor's office as well. This information can help prevent an unpleasant and unnecessary reaction to a prescribed medicine.

To sum it up, pharmaceutical companies that have developed patented products get a period of exclusivity when they can charge top prices. When the patent protection ends, other companies can compete with products that are the generic equivalent thus reducing the price.

After generic products have been on the market for a number of years with a proven record of efficacy and safety, manufacturers may then get FDA approval to manufacture and market essentially the same drug, with minor modifications, as a nonprescription, over-the-counter product. OTC drugs have a lower cost. In the next chapter you will learn all about OTC drugs and why they can save you a lot of money.

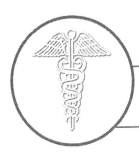

# FIVE

# OVER-THE-COUNTER DRUGS

The next step for some prescription drugs that have been on the market quite a while is for the FDA to consider them suitable for sale over the counter as a nonprescription product. Sometimes the dosage is reduced. Sometimes it isn't. The ailment the drug had been prescribed for no longer needs the supervision of a physician, and the new market for the product is considered enormous. There are a number of factors that come into play when the FDA decides to make a drug available over the counter, and sometimes it takes a couple of years, sometimes longer, and sometimes never.

Over-the-counter drugs can be real corporate moneymakers, a way for drug manufacturers to boost sales by offering a medication patients can self-prescribe when they experience any of a list of symptoms.

One of the best-known drugs to join the over-the-counter parade is Prilosec OTC, which had been one of the most commonly prescribed drugs for heartburn and acid reflux disease. Pharmacists say Prilosec is pretty much the same as Nexium, the highly advertised drug. You have probably seen the TV commercial: "The Purple Pill Called Nexium." (The same company, AstraZeneca, makes both products.)

When the company's patent for Prilosec ran out, Nexium was introduced for the high-cost brand name prescription market. Prilosec had its contents tweaked a bit and was sent to the huge over-the-counter market so AstraZeneca can have the best of both worlds—prescription and nonprescription.

But Prilosec and Nexium are not like a handy package of antacids to consume after dining on spicy Mexican food. Both Prilosec and Nexium are drugs that treat an ongoing heartburn and acid reflux condition. You have to buy them in fourteen-day supplies and take them daily until the supply runs out in order to calm down your acid reflux.

The Nexium and Prilosec packages advise (in small print) that if your heartburn continues to be a problem, you should contact your physician to find out if your stomach acid is a symptom of a more troubling ailment.

When Prilosec was first available, physicians in great numbers prescribed it. And it was expensive—more than $100 for a month's supply. Now you can get it as a nonprescription product for a lot less—unless you have prescription drug coverage that would have covered the original Prilosec prescription and now have to pay for Prilosec OTC because your plan covers only prescription drugs. It's quite backward. When it costs less—you have to pay more.

The FDA says there are more than eighty "therapeutic categories" of over-the-counter drugs, including products to treat acne, assist in weight control, relieve allergy symptoms, and cope with colds. An over-the-counter drug generally needs to meet several requirements, according to the FDA Center for Drug Evaluation and Research:

- The benefits need to outweigh the risks.
- The potential for misuse has to be low.
- Consumers have to be able to use it for a self-diagnosed condition.
- Labeling has to be adequate for instructing consumers how to use it.
- The monitoring of a health practitioner is not required for safe and effective use.

## How Do You Use Over-the-Counter Drugs?

You're sneezing, you're wheezing, your nose and eyes are red and watery. If you're like many people, you might say to yourself, "I'm suffering from my usual springtime allergies. Too much pollen in the air. I need some medicine to relieve my symptoms. Guess I'll pick up something at the drugstore after work."

Again, if you're like most people, you have little or no medical training, yet you are free to walk among the aisles at any pharmacy and fill your basket with a variety of medical remedies that contain active pharmaceutical ingredients. How do you know what to choose or if it will work for you? How do you know that medicating yourself is smart or safe?

Many people take recommendations from a friend. "Harriet's got the same kind of allergies as I do," you might reason. "She told me that she likes Claritin. It works fast, it does the job, and it doesn't make you drowsy." You buy it, you try it, and if your hunch is accurate, it works. Your symptoms let up, and you become one of the millions who not only use this over-the-counter drug but who recommend it to others.

That's what the manufacturer is hoping for. By making a version of the drug available to anyone, they expand their market. They may see it as a win-win situation for the consumer. A useful medication is made more widely available, especially to people who may not see a physician regularly, which benefits the company *and* the consumer, in their view.

But something else happened with the advent of the over-the-counter drug market. Insurance companies began dropping their coverage for drugs they used to pay for. Here's an example: One health plan used to include prescription-strength Claritin on its list of covered medications, so people were able to get the drug they needed for free or for a modest co-pay. When the medicine went over-the-counter, the company took it off their approved list, as the consumer could now purchase it at the drugstore without a prescription.

The problem was that the cost to the consumer went from a $10 to $15 co-pay to $45 retail for the same number of pills. Suddenly consumers were paying more money for a weaker medicine. (Not all OTC drugs are weaker than their prescription counterpart; check with your pharmacist.) Not only that, but many health plans dropped other prescription antihistamines from their list of covered drugs because they said patients could purchase an over-the-counter drug instead.

The Claritin story gets more complicated. It turns out that Schering-Plough, the company that created it, was about to lose the patent on the brand name drug. The generic form of Claritin, loratidine, would be available from generic drug companies; the medication would no longer be the sole property of its original manufacturer. So launching an over-the-counter version, which would capitalize on consumers' awareness of the original drug, made good business sense.

According to the May 2003 issue of *Drug Cost Management Report,* Wyeth's version of loratadine, Alavert, cost about 57 cents per tablet, and a thirty-day supply of the drug cost approximately $18. This compares favorably to the co-payment amount most plan members with a pharmacy benefit were paying for prescription Claritin. Members were paying anywhere from $16 to $35 for a thirty-day supply. However, if Claritin had remained available only by prescription, the journal reported, "the generic versions would likely be covered at the lowest co-pay level in most plans—less than $8 per prescription, on average."

*The New York Times,* also in May 2003, noted that the arrival of Claritin OTC had additional implications for similar drugs, and that the FDA might shift other prescription allergy medications, such as Allegra, Clarinex, and Zyrtec, to over-the-counter status—a move designed to reduce costs for consumers, but which might *increase* costs for some.

## THE POTENTIAL DANGERS OF SELF-DOSING

By the fall of 2003, concerns about the billions of over-the-counter drugs sold each year inspired the U.S. surgeon general to launch a television and print campaign to educate consumers about what they need to know about the medications they select for themselves.

The program, called "Be MedWise," was created to build awareness that over-the-counter drugs are powerful and must be used correctly to get full, safe benefits. Too often people were choosing the wrong drugs for the symptoms they experienced; some were taking the drugs in incorrect doses; and some were taking over-the-counter drugs that conflicted with other prescribed medications.

The campaign's commercials started airing in October 2003. At its Web site, www.bemedwise.org, you'll find advice on how to read a label, what parents should know before giving medicine to children, and how to avoid taking too much of an ingredient that may be in more than one medication.

The problem of overdosing on nonprescription, over-the-counter drugs is more than a simple concern—it's a serious medical crisis. A study published in the December 2002 *Annals of Internal Medicine* offered the shocking statistic that the number one cause of acute liver failure in the United States isn't cancer, alcoholism, or hepatitis. Nearly 40 percent of all patients diagnosed with liver failure had overdosed on acetaminophen, the most widely used nonprescription analgesic in the United States, and the active ingredient in the popular pain remedy Tylenol (and its many generic equivalents). How did this generally safe drug cause a life-threatening medical condition?

It turns out that acetaminophen can be dangerous when taken on an empty stomach or after drinking alcohol. Additionally, many people in the study had overdosed by taking more than one medicine that contained the drug as its active ingredient—for example, a couple of extra-strength Tylenol for a headache coupled with doses of a cold remedy that also contained acetaminophen. Though individual drug packaging is pretty clear about how much is too much, a lack of public awareness has added to the insidious nature of this serious health concern.

What can you do to protect yourself from developing a liver crisis? *Never* combine acetaminophen with alcohol; *never* take acetaminophen when you haven't eaten; *never* take more daily than the packaging suggests; and *never* take more than one medication that contains acetaminophen without first checking with your physician or pharmacist.

## A Smart Consumer Knows When to Ask for Help

An alert pharmacist is often the key to preventing serious medical problems from misuse of over-the-counter drugs. An October 2003 Associated Press article profiled Washington State pharmacist and geriatric specialist Stephen Setter, who reported that many families of Alzheimer's patients gave their "often agitated" loved ones Tylenol PM to help them sleep, not realizing that the medication contained an ingredient that might only add to the confusion of a patient with dementia. Setter also described an elderly patient who'd had a stomach ulcer but who took the painkiller ibuprofen, which caused stomach bleeding, when acetaminophen would have been a healthier and safer choice.

Do consumers really need a government education program about over-the-counter drugs? The FDA reports that more than 175,000 people are hospitalized each year because of misuse of nonprescription drugs. Some patients chose the wrong medicine, while others took more than the recommended dose. Again, it's worth mentioning that often people overdose because an ingredient is contained in more than one medication they're taking, but they don't realize it.

The National Council on Patient Information and Education commissioned a survey to discover how Americans self-medicate—what they think, what they know, and what they do. Since May 2002 most over-the-counter medicines have been required to carry a label containing "Drug Facts" to help consumers choose the best medication for their symptoms and understand how to take it with care. The council wanted to know how this educational labeling was working, and where additional effort was needed. The survey, a year after the "Drug Facts" label began appearing on over-the-counter medicines, discovered encouraging evidence that the labeling was a success. It found that:

- 56 percent of those polled were aware that this information existed.

- 44 percent of consumers consulted the label to find out the active ingredient in the medication product—up from 34 percent in a 2001 survey.

- 20 percent of consumers checked the label to learn about possible side effects from taking the drug—up from 10 percent in 2001.

- 23 percent checked the label to read dosage instructions—up from 16 percent in 2001.

However, 8 percent of buyers don't read the label at all. And almost half (48 percent) say they have taken more than the recommended dose of an over-the-counter medicine, convinced it will increase the effectiveness of the drug. Of these, 35 percent took the next dose sooner than they were supposed to, 32 percent took more than directed at a single time, and 18 percent took the drug more times a day than recommended.

Other problems the survey unearthed include combining medications (51 percent said they had taken both an over-the-counter and a prescription drug at the same time, which could result in too much of the active ingredient that was in both medicines), taking an over-the-counter medication for longer than recommended (44 percent), taking over-the-counter drugs instead of prescribed drugs (32 percent), and taking more than one nonprescription product that both had the same active ingredient (27 percent).

One of the most important findings of the survey was that many consumers did not speak with their health-care professionals before selecting over-the-counter drugs. More than 66 percent admitted finding the variety of available products confusing, but only 43 percent regularly consulted their pharmacists before purchasing nonprescription medicines. However, 80 percent said they would buy a specific over-the-counter medication if the pharmacist recommended it, and 82 percent said they would not buy a product if the pharmacist counseled them against it.

## How Can You Stay Safe on OTC Drugs?

It's one thing to accept a friend's suggestion of a restaurant or a travel destination. It's quite another to purchase medicine because someone at the office took it and got better quickly or because you saw an ad for it on television. If you're going to purchase and use over-the-counter drugs safely, be smart about it. The Be MedWise Web site "prescribes" asking plenty of questions about the drug you're planning to take.

### Talk to Your Pharmacist

Ask what drugs are available for the symptoms you need to treat. Ask how much you should take of the drug, how often you should take it, and when the best time is to take it. Ask how long it is safe to take it before checking with your doctor. Ask whether you should take it with food or liquid—or not. Find out if there are any medicines (prescription or over-the-counter), herbal products, dietary supplements, or vitamins that you should avoid while taking this drug.

### Read the Label

If you can't read the small print, use a magnifying glass or enlarge it on a photocopier. Read the *entire* label, especially the parts about potential side effects and "who shouldn't take this drug."

### Follow the Label's Instructions

With Prilosec OTC, for example, you won't get the full benefit of the product unless you complete the recommended fourteen-day treatment plan. Make sure you understand the instructions—and until you do, don't take the medicine.

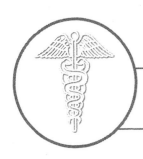

# SIX

# HERBAL REMEDIES, VITAMINS, AND MINERALS

Not every drug requires a prescription, as you've just read in the previous chapter, but taking these nonprescription medications requires you to be a careful consumer.

The same is true when deciding to dose yourself with something from the varied menu of herbal remedies, vitamins, and minerals that overflow on pharmacy and supermarket shelves. These products, sometimes known as *nutraceuticals*, come from many different manufacturers and a world map of countries. Because the FDA does not require them to be labeled as drugs, they may carry few if any warnings on their labels—and for the same reason, they don't have to meet the same rigorous testing requirements of prescription and nonprescription drugs sold to American consumers.

These bottles of herbals and vitamins, while offering promises of healing often at a much lower price than brand name or generic drugs, have the real potential to make you sick. They may also have the power to make you well, or at least to help the body heal itself.

While most of the products you'll find on store shelves are made with the best intentions, some may have dangerous side effects. Others can cause serious drug interactions with other medicines you may be taking. Still others don't make it clear how many pills you should be taking each day to get the promised result. And even when some do "prescribe" the appropriate dose, it's sometimes much larger than many in the medical community would encourage you to take.

What are these remedies, and what can they safely do for you? Who are your best sources for information about what to take and how to take it? How can you take reasonable precautions and still reap the benefits offered by these old-fashioned (in some cases) and newfangled (in others) products that in most cases are derived from exotic foreign plants, minerals, or even animal parts?

## WHY USE THESE PRODUCTS?

With the prescription drug prices sky-high, it's not surprising that consumers may succumb to the temptation to seek a less costly herbal product that promises a similar result. But saving money isn't a good enough reason to risk your health by jumping headlong into the "herb garden" without accurate information about what's available and how it works.

That's not to say that herbals must be avoided at all costs. Many herbal products, vitamins, and minerals may offer health benefits when used correctly. The challenge is to educate yourself about what each product can do for you, and then choose the most reliable manufacturer you can find.

The simple truth is that herbal products have been used for centuries by healers in many ancient and more recent civilizations. Herbs have been brewed into tea, made into poultices (dressings) to prevent infections, burned by Native Americans for their healing smoke, and crushed by mortar and pestle to make healing medicines.

Plants are the sources for many of our most valuable and powerful pharmaceuticals. This is one of the reasons for international concerns over the demise of the rainforest, which is where many of these growing "miracles" come from. Species of plants are disappearing at a disturbing rate from these tropical hothouses, and when they vanish, their potential as a source for future lifesaving medicines goes with them.

What kinds of plants go into making medicines? The heart medicine digitalis, for one, is derived from a plant called foxglove. Used correctly, it has saved thousands of lives. But readers of Agatha Christie mysteries know that when it's used by someone with murder in mind, it can be fatal!

## WHAT ARE HERBAL REMEDIES?

Walk down the aisles of any pharmacy, supermarket, or health-product store, and you'll find an astounding variety of herbal supplements, including:

- St. John's Wort
- Echinacea
- Ginkgo Biloba
- Saw Palmetto
- Yohimbe
- Evening Primrose Oil
- Glucosamine
- Shark Cartilage

The names are strange, but the promises on their packaging could not be more welcome. You see from the label that one bottle's contents may help you relax and sleep better. Another vows to help you fight off that nagging cold. Still another is the one your cousin Harry swears is the only thing that helped soothe his painful joints. And one suggests you use it instead of Viagra to boost your sex drive. It's all good news, right? Get a good night's sleep, enjoy sex more often, and stop sniffling all the time.

But what you don't know is that all of these supplements contain combinations of chemicals that may act on your body just as prescribed medication does. If you're already taking medicine for a chronic condition, an herbal product could interact badly with it. Even if you're popping an over-the-counter headache remedy, you could be harmed by introducing something else into your system.

"But," you argue, "why can I buy these products right off the shelf, no questions asked?" First, herbals are loosely classified as food supplements, as are vitamins and minerals, so they come under the jurisdiction of another part of the FDA. Second, each herbal on its own may not cause a problem. But when you have a medicine chest full of products for a variety of complaints, you may start taking a handful of pills each day—and the cumulative effect of these products may be bad for you. It's easier than you might think to take too much of a good thing.

## WHEN TOO MUCH CAN BE DANGEROUS

Vitamins and minerals are important to overall health. Your body needs vitamins and minerals in order to function properly, and unfortunately, we don't always get what we need from our diet. And sometimes we can get too much of one vitamin and not enough of another. Add up all those "fortified" cereals, dairy products, breads, and juices. Pile on a few "nutritious" meal replacement bars. Maybe you're taking one of those one-a-day, all-purpose vitamin/mineral pills in the morning—or for good measure, taking two of them! *It all adds up.*

Just about every manufacturer has jumped on the nutraceutical (trade name combining the words pharmaceutical and nutritional) bandwagon, making claims that its products deliver extra, added nutritional value. But then you actually start to add up what's on all the labels—beginning with the vitamins and minerals in a breakfast bowl of Total, for example. Should that serving of cereal replace your daily multivitamin pill? Check your bread wrappers and bottles of juice. More vitamins, more minerals. When is it all too much?

While it's difficult to overdose on most vitamins and minerals, it *can* happen. But becoming aware of what you're eating, drinking, and supplementing your food with is a good first step. Take iron, for example. It has been added as a supplement to a whole list of products, including breakfast cereals, fruit juices, breads—even soups. And, of course, it's in all the major multivitamin products you can buy in supermarkets and chain drugstores. With breakfast cereals, serving sizes are usually listed as "one cup." Most people eat as much as two cups every morning, which doubles the iron content. Add the natural iron contained in other foods, such as red meat, and it can really add up.

Can you overdose on iron? It depends. According to Marianne Ivey, Pharm. D., a professor at the University of Cincinnati College of Pharmacy, "too much iron can upset your stomach, causing constipation, and might interfere with the early detection of colon cancer." She says that older men and postmenopausal women in particular should be aware that too much iron could cause problems. "Because each individual has different needs for iron in their lives and has wide variety of diets," Dr. Ivey says, "you need to discuss your personal dietary needs with a physician who might advise cutting back a little on the iron or okay what you're taking."

## WHERE'S THE DANGER?

"People have been told that all these so-called natural, dietary products can't hurt you, and this is simply not true," says Mark D. Boesen, clinical pharmacist, the Apothecary Shops of Arizona. Some of the natural products that come from plants, the bark of trees, or minerals, Boesen says, can indeed hurt you. Ticking off a list of such dangerous items as hemlock (a deadly poison), cyanide (another poison), and cocaine (a dangerous drug and powerful stimulant), Boesen explains, "They're all natural too, but you wouldn't want to get near any one of them." He adds that just because a product is extracted from a plant doesn't necessarily make it safe for human consumption.

In a report entitled "Herbal Supplements, Consider Safety Too," the National Center for Complementary and Alternative Medicine said, "Just because an herbal supplement is labeled 'natural' does not mean it is safe, or without harmful effects. Example: The herb kava (or kava kava), a tension relaxer, [has] been linked to serious liver damage. A warning has been issued. FDA analyses of herbal supplements have found differences between what's listed and what's in the bottle. You may be taking more—or less—than what the label indicates."

For more information on herbal dietary supplements go to www.nccam.nih.gov/health/supplements.htm.

The October 2003 issue of *The New England Journal of Medicine* reported a study that checked more than 100 Web sites that were selling 115 herbal products known or suspected to contain aristolochic acid, an ingredient that has been found to cause cancer and kidney failure. These on-line herbal products had names such as Cold Away, Old Indian Herbal Syrup, Mother Earth's Cough Syrup, Cramp Relief, and PM-Ease. But neither the Web sites nor the manufacturers of these products told consumers what they needed to know.

How can this happen? Why aren't American buyers better protected from such dangers? These products don't come under close scrutiny by the FDA because they are classified as foods or food supplements not drugs. No clinical trials and tests are required to demonstrate that they work as promised, unlike what is demanded of prescription and over-the-counter drugs. What's even more surprising is that the safety and effectiveness of these nutraceuticals do not have to be documented.

Watchdog groups and individual citizens have been trying to get Congress to conduct hearings on this problem. The goal: to draft legislation that brings all herbal medications under FDA regulation as drugs. At the very least, proponents are demanding that herbal products contain package inserts that warn about possible drug interactions and overdoses. But just as with the pharmaceutical industry, the nutraceutical manufacturers exercise a lot of political power and are effective lobbyists in Congress. For now, you're unlikely to hear about changes in the laws affecting herbal remedies, so it's buyer beware.

## LEARNING TO USE HERBS AND VITAMINS SAFELY

That said, you should not completely give up on the idea of using herbals; some of these supplementary products may help you. Many of the more popular herbals have a wealth of anecdotal evidence that they deliver as promised. When individuals who aren't on other medications take them in moderate doses, they can be safe—and helpful. The key is being well informed about a product's risks and rewards.

"If you purchase herbal and other supplements in a health product store, or even in a supermarket that doesn't offer pharmacy services, you won't have the help of a pharmacist to advise you about potential dangers," *Smart Medicine*'s pharmacist advisor, Dr. Penna, says. "The clerks in these stores have not had any professional training and can only tell you 'we haven't had any complaints' or 'some of our customers swear by it.'"

Here's a terrific opportunity to seek professional advice from someone who should be up-to-date on the subject—your pharmacist. You'll learn more about how to do this in chapter 10, which covers "brown bagging"—bringing all your prescribed and over-the-counter drugs in for evaluation by your pharmacist. Don't forget to include all the herbal and vitamin-mineral supplements you are taking!

What kinds of problems might your pharmacist uncover with your basket of herbal remedies? According to the FDA report, it's all about interactions—the problems that occur when taking two medications that either work in opposition to one another or work similarly, dangerously increasing the potency. Suppose Marcia

## What Is Anecdotal Evidence?

The FDA requires many rules to be observed when pharmaceutical companies carry out clinical trials on human patients. This is one of the reasons that preparing a drug for market is so time-consuming and costly. The studies include people who take the as-yet-unapproved drug as well as people who receive only a placebo, a pill with no active medication. These tests are designed to get reliable evidence that any improvement in a patient's condition is due to the actual drug, not for any other reason (including positive thinking!). Often, thousands of patients will be studied before a drug can be sold by prescription.

But in the case of herbal remedies, the government doesn't require such testing, so the companies that produce these products don't do them. However, they may use people's success stories as part of their promotion of the product. Sometimes these stories come directly from the people who purchase the product on the recommendation of a friend or doctor; others are posted on Web sites or gathered by magazine and newspaper reporters. These "success stories" are called anecdotal evidence. No one has observed the person taking the product; no one has made certain it's been used correctly; and there's no way to check whether the improvement a person reports is due to any other factor, or if it occurred at all. It's simply an anecdote, a story about what someone has experienced.

The thing about anecdotal evidence is this: when enough people report that something works, word gets around. So when eight out of ten people who live in your senior housing complex insist that taking glucosamine and chondroitin sulfate pills have cured their aching joints so thoroughly they're running the New York City Marathon, taking tango lessons, or climbing Machu Picchu on their next vacation—it's difficult to ignore all those votes of confidence in the product.

is taking coumadin (a prescription blood thinner to prevent clotting), for example. Add to that the herbal supplement ginkgo biloba (her sister says it's good for keeping the brain sharp), aspirin (for a nagging sinus headache), and vitamin E (supposed to be good for resisting the effects of aging).

Another concern, according to the FDA, is combining a popular mood manager, St. John's Wort (see the box, "Take a Look at St. John's Wort"), with certain HIV drugs, which can significantly reduce their effectiveness. This widely used herbal supplement may also reduce the healing effect of prescription drugs for heart disease, depression, seizures, and certain cancers. St. John's Wort may even interfere with the reliability of oral contraceptives.

## Take a Look at St. John's Wort

What are the facts about this popular herbal remedy?

The Apothecary Shops of Arizona clinical pharmacist Mark Boesen says it can help with mild cases of stress and anxiety. In Europe, he notes, physicians regularly prescribe St. John's Wort for depression—while in the United States, you don't need a prescription for it because it is categorized as a dietary supplement. The active chemical is hypericum perioratum.

"St. John's Wort dates back to ancient times, when it was used for treating mental disorders," Boesen says. "But these days, if a patient suffers from more severe, longer-lasting depression, there are safer, more efficacious drugs to handle the situation. And if you're taking it as an insomnia remedy, it's recommended that you consider a safer drug, such as an over-the-counter antihistamine like Benadryl, which induces drowsiness as its significant side effect."

It's up to you to be a smart consumer of these products, and that means getting at the truth about any potential problems.

## VITAMINS

If you are taking any prescription, generic, or over-the-counter drugs, you need to inform your physician and your pharmacist about any vitamins and minerals you are taking. While vitamins in general are good for you and promote a healthy body, there are instances in which they can be harmful. This may sound shocking, but there are real reasons to be concerned about how they interact.

Margaret M. Gennaro, M.D., a physician associated with the Natural Horizons Wellness Center in Fairfax, Virginia, says you should be careful not to overdose with the fat-soluble vitamins A, D, E, and K. These vitamins don't wash away but instead accumulate in the body's fat deposits, which can be downright dangerous. All these vitamins can depress your liver function if ingested in high enough daily doses. If you're regularly taking medications along with herbal and vitamin products, your physician might want to order a liver function checkup.

An occasional overdose won't present that much of a problem, Dr. Gennaro says, but "it's when you are taking multiple vitamin pills, eating fortified cereals, and adding individual vitamins to the mix over a period of time that can cause problems." Dr. Gennaro recommends referring to *The A-Z Guide to Drug-Herb-Vitamin Interactions*, edited by Schuyler W. Lininger Jr. DC.

Some specifics to consider:

**Vitamin A.** Consuming too much vitamin A could cause headaches and changes in your eyesight. You might even turn a faint shade of orange if you oversaturate your body with this vitamin—by overeating carrots, perhaps. Women of childbearing years need to be especially careful because too much vitamin A can cause birth defects in a developing fetus. An overdose of vitamin A can also negatively affect bone density, making you more susceptible to developing osteoporosis. But at recommended dietary levels, vitamin A is very good for maintaining eye health. You just may be getting plenty from the food you're eating, so consider keeping track of how much vitamin A you ingest over the course of a week before taking a multivitamin or adding supplements.

**Vitamin B-6.** This water-soluble vitamin is important for red blood cell metabolism and helping keep your blood sugar level in a healthy range. Most people get plenty of this nutrient from their diets, because it's in fortified cereals, beans, meat, poultry, fish, and some fruits and vegetables. B-6 has at various times been recommended for carpal tunnel syndrome, premenstrual syndrome, and migraine relief, but the National Institutes of Health reports that no studies have successfully confirmed any of these claims. Very high levels of B-6 may cause nerve damage in your arms and legs. Check with your doctor to see what your B-6 levels are.

**Vitamin B-12.** This supplement is often mentioned as one that older adults should consider taking because their intestines may have been overrun by bacteria and yeast due to antibiotics and poor nutrition. If this is the case, older consumers should take a multivitamin pill with B-12. Or, if more might be needed, a physician can order a blood test to indicate how much you should take. The classic signs of B-12 deficiency are fatigue, numbness and tingling of the feet and hands, inability to concentrate, and depression. Check with your health-care professional to see whether you would benefit from either fortified foods or supplements.

**Vitamin C.** Some vitamins, such as vitamin C, are water-soluble. If you take too much of them, your body will usually flush the extra out when you urinate. But if you're popping more vitamin C than your body can easily excrete, you could develop kidney stones.

**Vitamin D.** This is the sunshine vitamin, and most people get what they need from casual exposure to the sun and perhaps a multivitamin. Usually milk is also fortified with vitamin D. Any other supplements are rarely needed, and too much vitamin D over time can cause deposits of calcium in soft tissues of the body, including the blood vessel walls and kidneys, where it can cause serious damage.

**Vitamin E.** Some authorities have recommended this vitamin, often sold in capsules of fish oil, to delay the development of heart disease. It also may protect against some forms of cancer and against many symptoms of aging. While certain foods (oils, nuts, some fruits and vegetables) supply vitamin E, many people don't get enough of this nutrient through food. If you choose to take a supplement, check the RDA (recommended daily allowance) on the package to be sure you aren't getting too much. Check with your physician to find out how much is too much for you.

**Vitamin K.** This vitamin can be surprisingly risky for anyone being treated for a heart ailment. Vitamin K can interfere with the effectiveness of blood-thinning (anticlotting) drugs such as Coumadin. You have to ingest quite a lot of vitamin K to reach a dangerous level, but it's definitely possible. Pharmacist Mark Boesen says that's why you should always talk to your physician and pharmacist about the foods you eat regularly and any vitamins you've been taking. If you consume a lot of broccoli and salad greens, for instance, you're getting large amounts of vitamin K. When this "dose" is added to your daily multivitamin and your daily bowl of fortified cereal, you may be getting enough to cause concern. Your doctor may decide to order a test that confirms you're getting the right amount for you.

What does all this mean? Most Americans should be able to get adequate vitamin support from a healthy and balanced diet. Unfortunately, all too many of us do not eat a healthy diet that is rich in such things as vegetables, whole grain bread, and fish products. If you eat a lot of fast food or even if you don't but you aren't getting the recommended three servings of vegetables and two servings of fruit a day, you should consider taking a daily vitamin pill as a safeguard. Taking megadoses of specific vitamins on top of your daily vitamins could be dangerous. Unless your physician specifically prescribes, or suggests, taking extra vitamins and minerals, it's not a good idea to do so.

# Food Guide Pyramid
## A Guide to Daily Food Choices

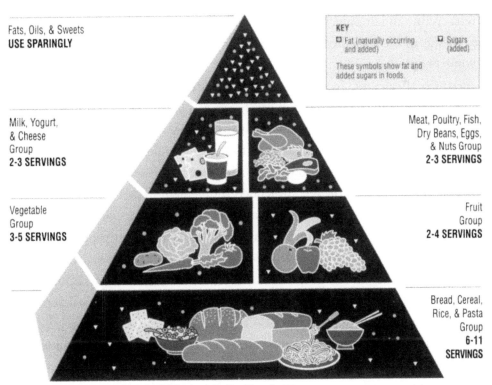

Source: U.S. Department of Agriculture/U.S. Department of Health and Human Services

## MINERALS

Minerals are an important nutritional component, and you can get most of what you need from a balanced diet. There are important exceptions, and if you're thinking of adding a mineral supplement for any of these reasons, make sure you're clear about what's healthy and what might do more harm than good.

**Calcium.** This nutrient is essential for your bones, and many people don't get enough from the food they consume. Options for getting the calcium you require include products designed as supplements or as osteoporosis prevention. You can even get additional calcium from popping a few Tums. Because calcium is not that easy a mineral for the body to absorb, you generally don't have to worry about overdosing. The excess calcium your body doesn't absorb is released when you go to the bathroom. Anything to worry about when it comes to calcium? Pharmacists suggest that when you're taking antibiotics such as tetracycline and doxycycline, do not also take extra calcium, which can weaken the potency of these medications. Also too much calcium can cause constipation in some people.

*Alert:* Coral calcium, an expensive and recently popular form of this mineral derived from the shells that make up coral reefs, is a poor choice. The FTC charged the marketers of Coral Calcium Supreme with making fraudulent and unsubstantiated claims that its product is designed to treat multiple sclerosis, heart disease, and cancer. It was also found to contain high levels of lead. Calcium carbonate, which costs much less, is the recommended supplement in this category.

**Iron.** Iron comes in two forms—one that is absorbed by your body when you eat meat, fish, and poultry. The other form, which occurs in plant products such as lentils and beans, is not as easily absorbed. This is one area where fortified products (flours, cereals, other grain products) can be a good idea. If you're not getting enough dietary iron, if you engage in regular intense exercise, if you're experiencing heavy menstrual periods, if you're a vegetarian—all of these can be valid reasons for supplementing with an iron pill. But too much iron can cause serious health concerns, so it's a good idea to confirm your iron status with your doctor before dosing yourself.

**Magnesium.** A National Institutes of Health fact sheet calls this "a mineral needed by every cell of your body" and notes that it helps maintain muscle and nerve function, and keeps heart rhythm steady and bones strong." Most people get their magnesium from nuts and green vegetables such as spinach, and deficiencies are rarely reported. A doctor can tell you if medical issues such as having diabetes or taking a diuretic means you should consider a magnesium supplement. Recent research suggests that higher levels of magnesium are linked to lowering blood pressure and decreasing risk of heart disease and post-menopausal osteoporosis, but results are incomplete. Important: Large doses of laxatives could cause a toxic level of magnesium, which can damage kidney function. Don't take a chance— check with your physician.

**Selenium.** This essential trace mineral is an antioxidant, and it has been suggested that low selenium levels can be linked to higher incidences of certain cancers. It has been suggested but not yet proved that selenium may help prevent symptoms of coronary heart disease; and some research has indicated that selenium can relieve symptoms of arthritis. So far, studies on all of these are inconclusive. Check with your doctor before taking a supplement, so that you don't chance an overdose.

**Zinc.** Zinc is vital for a healthy immune system. It helps heal wounds and maintain your sense of taste and smell. It's also important for normal growth and development during pregnancy, childhood, and adolescence. But zinc has also been touted as a "magical" mineral that can ease the discomfort of a cold and reduce its severity and duration.

The National Institutes of Health reports that a study of more than one hundred employees at the Cleveland Clinic indicated that zinc lozenges decreased the duration of colds by half, although no differences were seen in how long fevers lasted or the level of muscleaches. If this mineral is taken as recommended, 10 milligrams or so each day to reduce symptoms, it may do just that. But if you find yourself swallowing a couple of rolls of zinc lozenges one day, you could be at risk, especially if you're male. Men who exceed the recommended dosage, as much as 50 to 100 milligrams in a day, need to check with their physicians. According to the National Cancer Institute, large quantities of zinc contribute to the development of prostate cancer. A National Institutes of Health study of 47,000 men found that, compared with men who did not take supplements, men who took more than 100 milligrams of zinc a day had more than twice the risk of advanced prostate cancer.

If you're in the habit of piling on extra vitamins and minerals, you could be downing way too much of a good thing without realizing it. While the RDAs do change from year to year, they provide helpful guidelines to figuring out the optimum doses of these important nutrients. Read on to hear about some industry "wonders" that deserve to be carefully watched.

## SHOULD YOU HOP ON THE HERBAL BANDWAGON?

You often hear good things about the growing number of herbal products on drugstore shelves. How do you decide what's right for you? Pharmacist Mark Boesen provides an update on some of the most popular, with important health alerts you can't afford to ignore. Note that it is always important to talk to your pharmacist and physician before getting on a vitamin regimen since different people have different diets and require different dosages. Some vitamins can be harmful if you take too much for your body.

**Garlic.** Studies indicate garlic may help edge down cholesterol levels for borderline high levels. Patients with higher cholesterol usually respond better to a prescription medication. Note: Garlic may reduce the effect of blood pressure drugs such as cardizem and cardene and may increase the strength of drugs used to control diabetes. If you don't like the strong taste of garlic, you can take garlic pills instead.

**Ginkgo biloba.** This herbal product has been around a long time, and has been studied more than most herbal supplements. More than fifty clinical trials have been done, and research suggests it may help treat age-associated memory impairment and dementia, including Alzheimer's. Can it help improve memory and mental sharpness in all adults? The reviews are mixed, but it can be worth a try. Note: If you are taking a diuretic or other blood pressure control medication, check with your physician or pharmacist before using ginkgo biloba because it can negate the effectiveness of these hypertension drugs.

**Glucosamine and chondroitin.** Glucosamine naturally occurs in cartilage and connective tissue, but as people age, their bodies contain less of it. So does it make sense to take it in supplement form, along with its partner, chondroitin? Research indicates that this dynamic duo can promote cartilage repair and reduce deterioration, especially in the knees. Some twenty years of studies have backed up the efficacy of combining these two remedies. One important precaution: People with diabetes, or who might be susceptible to developing it, should be tested to make certain these supplements are not increasing sugar levels in the body. Many people who have diabetes are not aware of it. Everyone should be checked for this disease periodically, especially those who are overweight, inactive, or have a family history of diabetes.

**Echinacea.** This might be the "magic bullet" for the common cold. Or it might not. Many anecdotal claims exist that this supplement can help prevent colds or shorten their duration, but more studies are needed. In 2002 the National Institutes of Health funded a five-year, $6 million grant to build a botanical center in Iowa to research the potential of echinacea and St. John's Wort, so the next few years should produce more reliable evidence. Echinacea may interact with the anti-anxiety drug triazolem, making it more potent. Echinacea may also worsen the symptoms of autoimmune diseases such as rheumatoid arthritis.

**Kava (also called kava kava).** This dietary product is extracted from the root of a South Pacific plant. It's usually taken to cope with anxiety, relieve stress, alleviate tension, cure insomnia, and lessen menopausal symptoms. But the FDA warns that there is real risk of severe liver damage if you take too much of it.

**Milk thistle.** Anecdotal evidence suggests that milk thistle might help detoxify your liver, and it's currently part of a national research study for patients with hepatitis C. Milk thistle is a well-known herbal medicine that has quite a following. Ask your health store manager or pharmacist which products have the best quality ratings. The proper dosage usually comes in the package insert material.

**Saw palmetto.** This has been recommended for what have been called "benign" prostate enlargements, but many medical professionals believe that a urologist should supervise its use. Some evidence exists that it can inhibit testosterone, which can cause erectile dysfunction. One important consideration is if "benign" prostate concerns may be the beginnings of prostate cancer whether anyone should attempt self-treatment for such symptoms. Note: If you are already taking the prostate prescription drug finasteride (Proscar), saw palmetto might increase its potency to dangerous levels.

**Shark cartilage.** As the nation ages and more Americans suffer from damaged or overused joints, shark cartilage has been touted as a supplement that can help ease the pain. Boesen reports that "the notion that shark cartilage can promote human cartilage repair has never been clinically proven." Sharks are said to have lower incidences of some diseases (including cancer) than other mammals. But does that mean that ingesting shark cartilage will keep humans healthy? Dr. Carl Luer, senior scientist of the MOTE Marine Laboratory's Center for Shark Research in Sarasota, Florida, says no. "You have people catching and killing millions of sharks, grinding up their cartilage, and making misstatements to try to convince people that eating it will make them cancer-free," he says. "Unfortunately, there is no logical reason to conclude that freeze-dried shark cartilage pills taken orally could 'seek out' a malignant tumor in a cancer patient and inhibit the blood vessels feeding it." Also, he says, there is no reason to think that shark cartilage contains anything not found in other animal cartilage.

**Valerian.** This malodorous plant, used as a medicinal herb since the days of ancient Greece and Rome, is supposed to help ease anxiety and prevent insomnia. The results of numerous funded studies to date are inconclusive. Valerian, however, has been linked to liver damage when overused. There is no strict rule as to how much you have to take to become overdosed. It varies from person to person. Check with your physician on this, if you have any doubts. Some manufacturers may list a generally accepted dosage.

**Yohimbe.** This is a tree that grows in the African nations of Cameroon, Gabon, and Zaire, where for centuries it has been used as an aphrodisiac and sexual stimulant. It is a precursor for yohimbine, which must be prescribed by a physician. Does it actually enhance the male sex drive? Some evidence suggests it can, but unsupervised consumption of this drug can be dangerous, causing high blood pressure and abnormal heart rhythms. The prescribed product is safer because a physician supervises dosages.

## Can the Fruit of the Vine Heal Your Heart?

The scientific name for this natural remedy is oligomeric proanthocyanidin. In plain English, it's grape-seed extract, a powerful antioxidant.

Those who sell and promote it claim that the extract can help protect your blood cells from free-radical damage and that it can promote healthy circulation as a way to prevent cardiovascular disease. The essence of grape seeds is found in red wine. Europeans have long held that red wine can be good for the heart—one way or another. This seed extract is believed to be fairly safe, but it may interact poorly with cholesterol-lowering drugs such as Lipitor and Zocor.

## THE JURY IS STILL OUT

This chapter has profiled some of the most popular herbal remedies, as well as widely used mineral and vitamin supplements. There are many more. Their potential is intriguing, even exciting, but most also present problems if not carefully monitored.

You're much less likely to get into trouble if you follow what could be called the *Smart Medicine* mantra: Patient, physician, pharmacist. You, the patient, must keep your physician and your pharmacist in the loop: Make sure they know what herbal, vitamin, and mineral products you are taking so they can help you make sure you aren't overdosing or creating dangerous interactions.

The more prescription drugs you are taking, pharmacists say, the greater the potential for harm when you add supplemental products to the mix. A complete list of everything you are taking belongs in your patient medication profile on file at your neighborhood pharmacy (and your mail-order pharmacy, if you are using both).

Remember: Not everything for sale in a health products store, supermarket, or pharmacy is safe—even if it's all natural, your friends take it, and you read great things about it on the Internet.

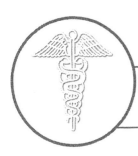

# SEVEN

# PRESCRIPTION MISTAKES: BE ON GUARD

Y ou've done it many times. Your physician diagnoses your condition, grabs a prescription pad, and scribbles out a prescription. More often than not, you can't read what's written, but you figure it must be some sort of clinical code. You take the prescription to your pharmacy and wait around for your medicine, or decide to come back later because the pharmacists are busy working on a backlog of orders. Maybe your physician or someone in the office phones in your prescription so you can pick it up later in the day.

This routine seems so simple; few patients realize that a lot can go wrong along the prescription communication pipeline. When something does go wrong, it can cost you a lot: time, money, maybe even your life. At the very least it can cost you the time of having the misread prescription refilled. In other instances it can cost you time and money if you are given the wrong prescription and have to pay for other medications to reverse the effects of the mistake. And in the worst case, the mistake may put you in the hospital or even cost you your life. Here are some possibilities of how things can go wrong:

- The wrong medicine, the wrong dosage, or the wrong dosage schedule may be written.

- The drug may not be appropriate for your age or disease.

- The drug may interact or add to the effect of a drug or supplement you are taking.

- The pharmacy may dispense the wrong drug or may misread the prescription or dosage.

## How Can Such Mistakes Happen?

First, your physician's handwriting might be the core of the problem. In a doctor's scrawl, the name of one drug might look a lot like another one. The pharmacist may misread it and misinterpret what was ordered. If that happens, you, the patient, could be in serious danger—because you took the wrong medicine or you took the right medicine the wrong way.

A study reported in the *Journal of the American Medical Association* in 2003 examined twenty-eight thousand Medicare enrollees to see how they fared with their medications. Of the adverse drug effects that were found to be very serious or fatal, 42 percent were deemed to be preventable.

In a case reported by the Institute for Safe Medication Practices in Huntingdon Valley, Pennsylvania, an elderly man was prescribed Minoxidil, a hair regrowth medication, four times a day. A mistranslation occurred, however, and by mistake the patient got Methotrexate, a rheumatoid arthritis and cancer medication. Methotrexate is only supposed to be taken once a week—certainly not four times a day. Although this mistake was caught in time, another elderly patient ended up dying after nine daily doses of Methotrexate.

The *FDA Consumer* magazine reported that many errors occurred in prescriptions for the arthritis drug Celebrex, the anticonvulsant Cerebyx, and the antidepressant Celexa. Fortunately, none of the more than one hundred reports of confusion among the three drugs has resulted in serious harm to a patient. In one case a physician wrote a prescription for "Celexa 200 mg." Because the antidepressant drug is available in only 20- and 40-milligram doses, the pharmacist called the doctor, who corrected his prescription to what he intended, the arthritis pain reliever Celebrex in a 200-milligram dose. Because of these and other such reports, the marketers of Celebrex, G.D. Searle & Co. and Pfizer Inc., have produced an educational ad campaign to alert health professionals to potential mix-ups.

The FDA's Office of Postmarketing Drug Risk Assessment carefully reviews the brand names of new medicines to avoid sound-alike and look-alike names. If the FDA believes that the name of a new product may be confusing to health-care professionals, the agency works with the drug company to rename the product.

## Mike Cohen, Prescription Watchdog

Pharmacist Michael R. Cohen, president of the Institute for Safe Medication Practices, has become an international watchdog whose organization spots and publishes all kinds of prescription medication errors. An advisor to the U.S. Food and Drug Administration, Cohen publishes a newsletter, *ISMP Medication Safety Alert!*, that digs up potential prescription errors and shows how to avoid them. Cohen received the Harvey A. Whitney Award from the American Society of Health-System Pharmacists for his lifetime work in spotting and eliminating prescription errors. For more information on current prescription errors and newsletter subscriptions, try the institute's Web site at www.ismp.org.

Here's the problem: Hastily written prescriptions can often be misunderstood and an entirely different medication dispensed. One of the early errors published by the Institute for Safe Medication Practices involved the special abbreviation language used by prescribers. The letter "U" stands for the word "units." According to the institute's spokesman, Chris Walsh, a person writing a prescription wanting to denote four units would write "4U." But with sloppy handwriting the "U" could end up looking like "0" and the instructions could be interpreted erroneously as 40 units. If a physician wrote "4U" for insulin, a medication that lowers blood sugar, and it was interpreted as 40 units, the person's blood sugar count could go too far down and cause hypoglycemia, a blood sugar so low it could become life threatening.

In another prescription handwriting mishap, a woman in her late fifties who was suffering from a dangerous blood-clotting condition was given a prescription for Coumadin (a blood thinner with the generic name warfarin). She was supposed to get 10 milligrams daily. But because the zero was unreadable, the dosage was read as 1 milligram. Here the danger was not from overdosing but underdosing. Two weeks after she was prescribed this medication to thin her blood, the woman suffered severe blood clots in her legs—one of the clots could have broken, gone to her heart.

Edward J. Staffa, a pharmacist who works with the National Association of Chain Drug Stores, gives some examples of drugs that look and sound very much alike:

**Fiorinal and Florinef.** Fiorinal, a pain reliever, looks and sounds like Florinef, which is a hormone. These drugs produce such different effects on a patient that an accidental switch could cause considerable harm.

**Lomotil and Lamictal.** Lomotil is for diarrhea, and Lamictal is for epilepsy. A switch in these two medications, he says, could create all kinds of havoc.

**Plendil and Isordil.** Plendil slows down the heart, and Isordil improves blood flow, thus speeding up the heart.

## PRESCRIPTION E-SCRIBING

Technology has already provided valuable safety options for consumers. Some electronic prescription writing services, such as Express Scripts and OnCallData, are turning up in physicians' offices. They provide the means of sending prescriptions electronically, eliminating the handwriting problem.

But according to an October 2003 Associated Press article, doctors concerned about the expense of being required to write Medicare prescriptions electronically are asking lawmakers for help, and it looks like they may be getting it. A clause in the new Medicare bill provides for grants to help defray the costs of e-prescribing.

"Ultimately, it's costly for patients. Initially, it's costly for the physicians," said Senator Jon Kyl of Arizona. He and others are opposed to making the electronic prescription program mandatory, saying it's too early to insist on the new way of transmitting prescriptions.

"The technology is ready," says Barrett Toan, chairman of Express Scripts, one of the pharmacy benefit managers asking Congress to support the program. Under the electronic program being proposed, a physician would connect to a database via the Internet and get information about a patient's other prescriptions, any potential negative drug interactions, and even suggestions for generics and low-cost brand name alternatives. However, to transmit such sensative information requires expensive software that ensures security.

In their original Medicare bills, lawmakers on both sides of the Capitol included an e-prescription program—with the House asking that it be mandatory by January 1, 2006, and the Senate keeping it voluntary but offering a program of physician grants to help purchase the technology.

Medical societies such as the American College of Physicians and the American Medical Association urged their members to write their representatives and express opposition to the mandatory program, even going so far as to offer a sample letter on their Web sites. Their concerns seem to be mostly financial, but Toan insisted that the software and upgrades will cost physicians much less than early reports said. For now, the program is voluntary.

## Ask the Prescriber

It all starts in your doctor's office. Or your dentist's office, or any other prescriber's office where prescriptions are written or phoned in to a pharmacy. Any time you visit a prescriber's office with a problem that requires drug therapy, you should bring along a notepad and a pen. Write down the name of the medication your doctor is prescribing, along with the dosage and dosage schedule. It makes good sense to ask questions when a prescription is in the works. You need to fully understand your diagnosis and get the information you need from the pharmacist who will fill the prescription.

"Don't accept an unsafe prescription," says Eleanor M. Vogt, pharmacist and Senior Fellow Ph.D. with the Institute for the Advancement of Community Pharmacy, based in Alexandria, Virginia. "It's unsafe," Dr. Vogt says, "if you can't read it. If you have trouble reading it, so might a pharmacist, who, in a hurry, might interpret the handwriting incorrectly, and you could get a potentially dangerous medication."

Once, as a patient, Dr. Vogt received a prescription that she could not read from a physician. She says, "He told me not to worry, the pharmacist could read it, and I told him 'I'm a pharmacist, and I can't read it.'" Embarrassed, the physician then carefully printed out the prescription.

Sometimes busy physicians may be a little annoyed at having their handwriting second-guessed. "It's your right," Dr. Vogt points out, "and they generally go along with it." As well they should. That sloppily written prescription could come back to haunt them if a patient suffers an injury from a prescription that was dispensed in error because of unclear handwriting.

"After insisting on getting a prescription you can read," Dr. Vogt says, "make sure that the purpose of the medication is included." This is vitally important because if a mix-up occurs in the name of the drug, knowing why it was prescribed will help clear things up. For instance, the prescription should indicate that the medicine is for controlling blood sugar, lowering blood pressure, soothing itchy skin—whatever ails you. This way, you won't be getting a look-alike or sound-alike product by mistake.

Always take notes when you visit any office where prescriptions are written for you. Get the name of the medication being prescribed, what it's for, how it should be taken, how long it should be taken, and any potential side effects. Ask your physician if this medication requires any special monitoring tests, such as those given to check blood pressure, blood sugar, kidney function, or liver function. Don't leave until you've been fully informed by your physician about what to expect from this medication. It's your right—and your responsibility. Remember the mantra: *Physician, Pharmacist, Patient.*

## At the Pharmacy

Now you're at the pharmacy. You have your prescription in hand (or perhaps it has been phoned in). By law you have the right to medication counseling, and it won't cost you a dime. *Take advantage of it.* Don't just accept the prescription and depart. Sometimes a clerk will ask you to sign a paper that says you waived the right for consultation. *Don't sign.* It may take a few more minutes to wait until the pharmacist is free and available to talk with you. But it's worth the wait, especially if there is anything about taking the medicine that you don't understand.

Make sure you're told what the medicine is for and what it will do. Here's where a mix-up can be detected quickly, if what's being described is not what you're being treated for. This is a final step, a last chance to make sure you are getting the right medication, in the right doses, and with the right timing.

At this point, if you haven't done it before, it's a good idea to show the pharmacist your list of the drugs you are taking, including any nonprescription remedies. If you've already set up a patient profile with this pharmacy, ask the pharmacist to have it available during the consultation.

Review the bottle label with the pharmacist to make sure you understand the dosage—when and how you are supposed to take the medicine. It's even a good idea to open the prescription box and check what's inside to make double sure you're getting what was ordered and to take a quick look at the package insert (which contains instructions and warnings) to see if you have any other questions.

Maybe the pills don't look like the ones you've been taking. This could point to a mistake or it could simply be that the color or shape changed when the product went from a patented brand name to a generic drug manufactured by several companies.

Also take a look at the bottle or box that will go into your medicine cabinet. Make sure the name of the drug and what it's for is recorded on the label. Later, when it's sitting on the shelf, you'll need to be able to quickly identify it and know what the medicine is for. This is especially important if you are taking the medication only "as needed."

With refills, you won't need another consultation, but you should double check the information on the box and the bottle inside to make sure it's *your* medication and *not* something else. Open it up and see what's inside. Mistakes like this are rare. But, packaging mishaps do happen. Also, make sure your name is on the prescription and not somebody else's.

## What If the Pharmacist Isn't There?

For patients ordering online or by mail, there's a different drill. You have the right to get the same kind of counseling with a pharmacist as you get at your neighborhood pharmacy. When you place your order, be sure to let the pharmacist at the other end know about all the drugs you are taking—prescription and over-the-counter—to make sure you won't be harmed by a bad mixture. Of course, this holds true in reverse. Your local pharmacist should be aware of any on-line drug purchases you may be taking.

Keep everyone up to date on what you're taking. If you're having prescriptions filled locally and from a distance, make sure all your pharmacists know what drugs you are taking. Both places should have your complete list of drugs, so you never end up with medicine that may interact dangerously with the other drugs in your medicine cabinet.

## THE HOSPITAL SCENE

If you are being treated in a hospital, you could be getting new drugs that interact poorly with other medicines you have been taking. That's one of the reasons most hospitals insist you do not "self dose" while you are a patient there, including over-the-counter remedies like acetaminophen or ibuprofen. If you have any allergies or concerns about drug interactions, you must supply the hospital staff with complete information.

Here is where you need a patient advocate, someone with a list of drugs you have been taking who can double check any pills and liquids you're given by hospital staff. You may be groggy during treatment, which means you may accept anything handed to you by a nurse at your bedside.

Your advocate can be a family member or a friend. It's ideal to have someone with you in the hospital as much as possible. If necessary, a pair of advocates can relieve each other.

Remember that it's your right to ask the nurse what you are being given before it is administered. Ask to speak with the hospital pharmacist if the nursing staff can't answer questions to your satisfaction.

Your physician (or physicians, if more than one is involved in your hospital care) should list on your chart all medications you will be taking. Make sure that these prescription names (and any nonprescription drugs that may be indicated) are listed on the clipboard at the end of your bed. You or your patient advocate should check to see that it is up to date. And ask whoever is dispensing medications for you to check the chart to make sure you are not getting a medicine that someone else was supposed to get.

Dr. Penna suggests you should be asking the same questions you ask your regular physician. What is the medicine, and why was it prescribed? When a nurse walks in with a syringe or a paper cup containing a pill, you want to know what it's for and whether it matches what's on your chart.

Why should you be so careful and conscious about the medications you are given in the hospital? According to a report—"To Err Is Human"—published by the Institute of Medicine in 2000, more than 14,000 hospital patients die each year from drug mix-ups in hospitals. Another 750,000 experience severe drug interactions but survive. Half of these prescription calamities in hospitals are caused by drug side effects, while the other half are caused by the patient getting the wrong dose or medication.

In the September/October 2000 issue of *FDA Consumer* magazine, the American Hospital Association listed some of the most common medication errors:

- Incomplete patient information (not knowing about patients' allergies, other medicines they are taking, previous diagnoses, and lab results, for example)

- Unavailable drug information (such as up-to-date warnings)

- Miscommunication of drug orders, which can involve poor handwriting, confusion between drugs with similar names, misuse of zeroes and decimal points, confusion of metric and other dosing units, and inappropriate abbreviations

- Lack of appropriate labeling when a drug is prepared and repackaged into smaller units

- External factors, such as lighting, heat, noise, and interruptions, which can distract health professionals from their medical tasks

By participating actively in your care while in the hospital, you can do much to prevent becoming a victim of medication mistakes. You and your patient advocate can provide a checkpoint past which the wrong pills or doses may not go.

## You're the Manager

When it comes to sorting out all the different prescription and nonprescription products you are taking, you have to be the manager. If you are incapacitated, then it becomes the responsibility of your designated patient advocate, whether a family member or a friend, to monitor the drugs you are taking. (Designate someone

## It Happens Even at the Best Hospitals

It was possibly the most widely reported drug overdose in history. A patient who was part of an experimental breast cancer drug study received four times the already-high prescribed dose of the chemotherapy drug cyclophosphamide over a four-day period. For two months, her physicians didn't even realize that the overdose had caused the patient's death.

Why did this error capture so much attention? The patient was Betsy A. Lehman, a thirty-nine-year-old health columnist for the *Boston Globe*, and the hospital was the world-famous Dana-Farber Cancer Institute. Stories about this medical nightmare appeared in major media, and it became a cautionary tale at medical conferences all over the world.

In an interview in the October 2001 issue of *Medical Economics*, Martin J. Hatlie, president of Partnership for Patient Safety and a leader in preventing medical mistakes, said, "The reaction within medicine was: If such a preventable error can happen at an institution like Dana-Farber, it can happen anywhere." But, he added, "Celebrated failures often spark change, and this, coupled with the wrong-leg amputation case in Florida a few months later, became patient safety's Chernobyl. The Lehman case helped lead to the recognition that medical errors are most often caused by system-wide failures rather than by an individual who goofs."

At the time, a *Boston Globe* editorial accused the hospital of failing to notice an error "so glaring that any first-year medical student should have spotted it." A columnist wrote that the overdose errors "would make The Three Stooges look like brain surgeons," and described the mistakes as "nothing less than criminally negligent homicide."

What actually happened to cause the fatal overdose?

In the fall of 1994, Dana-Farber was using an experimental protocol with women whose breast cancers were not responding to traditional treatments. The protocol being tested used high doses of cyclophosphamide in conjunction with cimetidine and stem-cell transplants.

In the middle of November, a research fellow on the team apparently misread the protocol and by mistake ordered four times the correct dose of the chemotherapy drug for Lehman and another patient, according to court documents. Lehman experienced a severe reaction but recovered and was about to be discharged when she suddenly died. The other patient suffered severe toxicity and was transferred to an intensive care unit but survived. She died two years later of breast cancer.

The overdoses weren't discovered until February 1995, and the facts of what happened are still being disputed. Apparently, some members of the team questioned the size of the dosage but didn't prevent it from being administered in large part because of assumptions that others had already said it was correct.

According to news reports, the patient's family received a confidential settlement from Dana-Farber described as a "multimillion-dollar sum" to satisfy a wrongful death suit. In addition, officials at Dana-Farber instituted corrective measures and new policies dedicated to patient safety.

you trust for this important role—*before* you get sick.) The more medicines you take, the greater the danger you can be in. You need to become an instant expert in the medicines you are taking. But don't despair: Many resources are available. Your medical team—physician, pharmacist, and nurse—can help, but you can do some research on your own.

*Medication Errors*, a book published by the American Pharmacists Association, is aimed at health-care professionals, but it's definitely worth a look. Check at your library, or you can order it through the Institute for Safe Medication Practices at Web site www.ismp.org. The institute also offers a pamphlet on how to use medications safely and another on what to do in the hospital, at the doctor's office, and at home.

You can order *Your Medicine: Play It Safe*, a booklet published by the National Council on Patient Information and Education in conjunction with the federal Agency for Healthcare Research and Quality, directly from the government by calling (800) 358-9295. Request publication #03-0019.

# UNDERSTANDING YOUR PHARMACIST

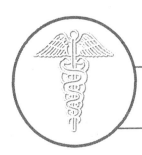

# EIGHT

# MEET YOUR PHARMACIST

Too many consumers have grown up with an incomplete understanding of what happens behind that counter in the local drugstore. They've viewed pharmacists as educated clerks whose primary function is to decipher the chicken scratching of doctors' handwriting, fill small bottles of pills from bigger bottles, and type up labels to identify each prescription dispensed.

These preconceptions may come from years of viewing old movies, where the kindly small-town druggist also scoops ice cream cones, recommends remedies for an aching back, and provides sage advice on subjects ranging from unrequited love to the croup.

Don't believe everything you see in the movies. Times have changed, the medical field has grown more complex with each year, and the job of the pharmacist has evolved along with it. In this chapter, you'll learn just how valuable a partner in self-care your pharmacist can be.

## WHAT GOES ON BEHIND THE COUNTER?

Here's the scene repeated daily in pharmacies all over the country: Sandra, a regular customer, stops in to pick up a prescription. She hands the signed prescription slip to a woman at the counter, who tells her it will take about twenty minutes for her medicine to be ready. While she is waiting, she walks up and down the aisles, where she adds to her shopping basket an over-the-counter remedy for her husband's nagging heartburn, a bottle of acetaminophen (on sale) to keep in her desk at the office for occasional headaches, and a birthday card for her niece. As she passes the prescription pick-up counter on her wanderings around the store, she can see people working back there.

Most wear white jackets, but not all. Some appear to be consulting computer screens while others are talking on the telephone. Still others are searching shelves for large containers, which they bring over to a worktable on the side to prepare a prescription.

In some pharmacies, a customer may be invited to join the pharmacist in a small booth for a private consultation away from others waiting to be served. Sandra may overhear a bit of a conversation about renting or buying a home blood pressure monitor.

The pharmacy staff members working behind the counter have different jobs and varied training to prepare for them. The senior members are licensed pharmacists, and under them are pharmacy technicians, specially trained employees who assist pharmacists. Some busy pharmacies also employ cashiers who ring up your bill but must refer your questions to someone else.

Let's meet these people and discover why they're permitted to dispense prescription drugs, advise customers on when and how to take their medication, and provide information about other health-care resources they may want or need.

## WHAT'S A PHARM.D.?

These days, pharmacists must spend almost as much time on their studies and training as physicians. Their coursework includes pharmacology, chemistry, the pharmaceutical sciences (the study of drug behavior in the body), and the social sciences. Pharmacy students are also required to serve internships, where they get plenty of hands-on training in neighborhood pharmacies, as well as in hospitals, nursing homes, and clinics. They are constantly trained in how best to communicate with patients and other health-care professionals. This patient-relationship work is practiced and graded over and over again.

Pharmacists must complete a specialized four-year course of study in a college, university, or school of pharmacy. (Entry requirements for all colleges and schools

# Who Becomes a Pharmacist, and How?

Let's take a look at three people considering the profession of pharmacist.

### DIANA – DECIDING ON PHARMACY

Diana loves her high school science classes, and so when she arrives at the University of Wisconsin, Madison, she is thinking about premed. But a careful reading of the university Web site has pointed her toward a pharmacy program. She'll need to take two years of pre-pharmacy coursework to qualify for the program. Inorganic and organic chemistry, calculus, physics, even zoology is on the list. Plus English, economics, ethnic studies, sociology, and more—a thorough liberal education with a strong science emphasis, before she even begins her professional studies. That includes plenty of hands-on lab work, as well.

### MICHELLE – APPLYING FOR PHARMACY SCHOOL

Michelle completed the necessary science and general education requirements as an undergraduate at the University of Illinois, but she wasn't sure about her career choice until she spent some time chatting with the new pharmacist in her hometown. She liked the idea of working in a helping profession, she hoped to start a family in a few years and found the schedule appealing, and she was intrigued by the constantly evolving drug plans of treatment for her grandmother's breast cancer.

Michelle decided to apply for a doctor of pharmacy program at the University of Illinois, Chicago. On the Web site, she studied the planned coursework for the four-year program. It included:

**FIRST YEAR**

Fundamentals of Drug Action I & II
Human Physiology and Pathophysiology I & II
Drug Delivery Systems I & II
Pharmacokinetics

**SECOND YEAR**

Fundamentals of Drug Action III & IV
Drug Delivery Systems III & IV
Principles of Drug Action and Therapeutics I–IV
Contemporary Pharmacy Practice
Pharmacy Systems Management
Drug Information and Statistics
Social and Behavioral Pharmacy

**THIRD YEAR**

Principles of Drug Action and Therapeutics V–VIII

Pharmacy Law

Pharmacy Services and Reimbursement

Nonprescription Pharmaceuticals and Herbal Medicinals

Principles of Pharmaco-economics and Drug Treatment Outcomes

**FOURTH YEAR**

Students will serve seven clerkships, four in Ambulatory Care, Hospital, Community Practice, Medicine. The other three are elected from these choices: Administrative, Geriatric, Advanced Ambulatory Care, Home Health, Community Practice, Kinetics, Advanced Medicine, Nutrition, Pediatric, Critical Care, Psychiatry, Drug Information, Surgery.

Michelle took a deep breath. It was an amazingly thorough program, with coursework and clerkships (like internships) in all kinds of settings where she might choose to work in the future. She could see that earning a doctor of pharmacy degree could be as demanding as going to medical school.

## SCOTT – FINISHING PHARMACY SCHOOL

Scott is just about to graduate from pharmacy school in Maryland and is looking eagerly toward starting his career as a pharmacist in his home state of Delaware. He received excellent grades as an undergraduate and when he meets with his advisor, he finds out what else is required of him before he can begin to practice.

First, he must fill out an application for licensure with the Delaware Board of Parmacy, which regulates the practice of pharmacy in that state. Second, he must provide evidence that he has graduated from a college or school of pharmacy that is accredited by the American Council on Pharmaceutical Education, the agency that reviews and approves all colleges and schools of pharmacy in the U.S. And finally, he must pass the North American Pharmacist Licensure Examination and the Multistate Pharmacy Jurisprudence Examination.

of pharmacy vary, but most require at least two years of undergraduate work.) Many pharmacists earn a Bachelor of Science degree, then complete four years at a professional pharmacy school, after which they earn the degree of doctor of pharmacy (Pharm.D.). This course of study is similar to that of dentistry and medicine. Like physicians, pharmacists must learn to care for patients with many different requirements and in all kinds of health-care environments.

Most pharmacists work closely with physicians during their studies, and some universities now require medical students and pharmacy students to enroll in the same courses. Requiring a similar education for physicians and pharmacists certainly will benefit their future patients. They should be equally well informed about the latest pharmaceutical research and able to team up in providing the best possible medical care.

The learning doesn't stop when a pharmacist completes a degree. All pharmacists must take fifteen hours of continuing education every year so they can keep up with the constant infusion of new drugs, learn about familiar drugs now being prescribed for other ailments, and be alerted to possible problems affecting commonly prescribed medications.

## WHAT DO PHARMACISTS KNOW?

As we've just seen, pharmacist training is rigorous and comprehensive. These days, your neighborhood pharmacist will have completed coursework in:

- Drug chemistry
- The systems of the body down to the cellular level
- How drug dosages are calculated and how drugs are metabolized by the body
- How to function in a professional manner with patients.
- How drugs are researched and designed
- How drugs act on the body and the brain
- The pharmacist's role in wellness and disease prevention
- How alternative medicines and nutrition affect prescription drugs
- How to evaluate, monitor, and counsel patients
- How to manage personnel in various settings
- How to review professional literature, pharmacy, and the law (federal, state, and regional regulations and distribution)
- How to work in managed-care systems

- How the health needs of men and women differ

- How to integrate knowledge of chemistry, pharmacology, and toxicology when it comes to treating pain and substance abuse

Doctoral students even learn about nonprescription pharmaceuticals and herbal medicines, so they can successfully perform the pharmacist's role as educator and advisor to patients.

A pharmacist's education is extensive and exacting. But that's not the entire story. Pharmacists are licensed and responsible for products with the power of life and death. Professional ethics demand that every pharmacist consider the safety and the well-being of patients their top priority.

## What Can a Pharmacy Tech Do?

But pharmacists can't do it alone. Most pharmacies employ pharmacy technicians, who are required to complete a challenging and specific training to properly assist the pharmacist and the patient-customer.

Mission College in Santa Clara, California, offers an intensive twenty-one-week program for aspiring pharmacy technicians. Classes are mostly in the evening, which lets students work full time while acquiring the knowledge and skills to be licensed as pharmacy technicians by the California State Board of Pharmacy. This training program, like many others in different states, provides approximately three hundred hours of instruction, both in theory and in practical, hands-on

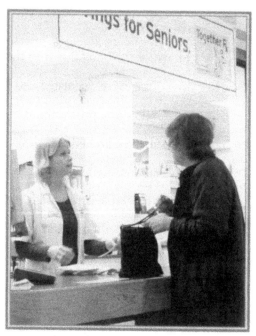

*A Ukrop's pharmacist helps a customer.*
Photo courtesy of Ukrop's

training. Students are also required to serve what's called an externship, where they work outside the program under supervision to gain pharmacy tech experience for anywhere from 120 to 240 hours.

To qualify for such a program, students must:

- Pass assessment testing
- Go through a formal interview
- Have a high school diploma or GED
- Pass a drug test
- Have no criminal background
- Type at least twenty words per minute
- Demonstrate strong English, math, and communications skills

## What Does a Pharmacy Tech Training Program Prepare People to Do?

At Mission, students learn about pharmacy practice and about successful communications (both verbal and nonverbal), conflict resolution, human relations, customer service, and patient confidentiality issues. They are trained in pharmacy terminology and abbreviations, the identification and use of pharmaceutical and medical terms, and abbreviations and symbols common to prescribing and dispensing medications.

They'll also study the preparation, properties, uses, and actions of drugs; learn the brand and generic names of drugs and classifications; and develop skills in reading all kinds of medical labels. Students will practice "pharmacy math," which relies heavily on fractions, ratios and proportions, and conversions for drug calculations. They will learn to calculate common dosage determinations by using a variety of approaches involving metric, household, and apothecary measurements.

Here's a sample of what pharmacy tech students learn:

- How to operate over-the-counter health-care devices and train patients in using them.

- How to identify supplies and devices needed by patients with chronic diseases such as diabetes.

- How to aid people coping with surgical procedures that have resulted in ostomies (an operation to create an artificial passage for waste elimination).

- How to process prescriptions and keep records using computer-based systems.

## M.D. MEETS PHARM.D.

Pharmacists frequently have the information you need and the answers you want when it comes to nonemergency medical concerns. Pharmacists can save you a lot of money on the drugs by suggesting lower-cost generic products or even over-the-counter remedies that could basically produce the same results. Pharmacists can also ensure that one of your doctors has not prescribed a medication that interacts badly with other drugs you are taking. It's a common problem, which can make you sicker and cost you even more money.

But how can your pharmacist act as your "purchasing agent" to help you get the best medicine at the best price? And what can your pharmacist do as your "safety monitor" to make sure your medicine cabinet doesn't become a dangerous place?

You'll learn the answers to both those questions in chapter 9, "Take Your Pharmacist to Lunch." But the first step in partnering with your pharmacist can be introducing your doctor (or assistant) to your pharmacist. Facilitating that kind of connection can help you get the right medicines at the right price, the pharmacist may benefit from referrals, and the physician strengthens the patient relationship.

It may not be easy to make this happen. Your physician may be too busy to chat with your pharmacist, and it may take awhile to get the physician's staff assistant to work with you. Provide the assistant the pharmacist's phone number and the pharmacist the physician's. If the pharmacy is located close to the physician's office, they may already be in touch. (If you don't have a regular pharmacy, consider asking your doctor's staff for a recommendation.)

If this sounds like a pipe dream that is unlikely to happen, think again. It's a proven, professional strategy used by major clinics and medical centers such as

Kaiser Permanente, which recommends that its physicians and pharmacists communicate with each other if there is any question about a medicine's efficacy or cost. Kaiser's goal is simple: It wants the best health outcomes for its patients, and it doesn't want to spend any more money than necessary.

Consider this scenario: Your physician diagnoses your condition and then starts writing a prescription. This is when you should ask about the cost. If that sounds rude or inappropriate, it shouldn't. You're the one footing the bill for the physician and the prescription. Does the physician know of any other medicine that might work just as well but comes with a lower price tag? You might be surprised that many physicians have no real idea what a particular medication will cost.

This is the moment to provide your friendly pharmacist's number. Your physician or a staff person can discuss whether there is an equivalent medicine at a better price. This type of conversation provides medical case management with your best interests at its core. Your physician may not know all the details of your patient profile, especially if you see more than one doctor for your different needs. By asking for your doctor's help in getting the best price for a needed prescription, you're demonstrating that you're actively involved in your health care. By involving your pharmacist in the discussion, you're using your medical resources to best advantage.

But what if your physician phones in a prescription after you've left the office? You go to the counter and ask the pharmacist how much it's going to cost. If the price makes you gasp, ask if a lower priced, equivalent product is available. If so, then you might ask the pharmacist to phone your physician to see if a switch can be made.

As a rule doctors' offices make a real effort to respond to calls from pharmacists. But be prepared to wait. Both your physician and pharmacist are busy people and may prefer to make and take phone calls at specified times during the day.

## WHAT THE PROS SAY

"When the price is too high for a patient," says Barry Tompkins, a pharmacist in Fulton, New York, "I call the doctor and ask about trying some therapeutically equivalent product that costs less." It's important, Tompkins adds, that people understand how the system works when they want their pharmacists to ask physicians whether it's possible to change prescriptions. "Officially, the patient has to ask for help with the cost, because ethically we can't tell the patient to get another drug that the physician hasn't prescribed," he says.

Here's how it goes: You ask your pharmacist about the cost of your medicine and if another product would provide the same effect at a lower cost. Tompkins describes it as "a little dance you have to do." Maybe, over time, your various physicians and your newfound pharmacist friend can brainstorm together *before* a prescription is written to make sure you get the right medication at the best possible price.

Pharmacist Larry Oliver in Athens, Alabama, says he frequently provides customers with prescription costs before the medicine is dispensed. Oliver echoes Tompkins in noting that the patient has to ask for help before the ball starts rolling to get a better price. Some physicians get grumpy about being bothered with calls from pharmacists, Oliver notes, but he says most are open to suggestions. And why not? Paying less for a prescription makes their patients' lives easier, and it costs little besides a few minutes of their time to make it happen.

Kristin E. Thomas, M.D., former chief resident at Johns Hopkins University Hospital in Baltimore and currently in private practice, comments, "Some doctors are nervous about working with pharmacists because they don't really know who they are and what they really do. When a pharmacist calls to suggest another medication that costs less for the patient, some doctors might not like the appearance of being challenged. In our practice, we have good, working relationships with some twenty pharmacies in our area."

More often than not, Dr. Thomas adds, she will go along with a pharmacist's suggestion. But in some cases a higher-cost product is called for because of the patient's medical history and special needs. She cites the following case:

The patient's LDL cholesterol level was way too high and needed to come down. Instead of using the less costly product at the time, I wrote a prescription for another drug, which costs more because we had to 'power down' the LDL number and the patient would have needed too high a dose of the less expensive product.

This is a good example why it's important that your physician mentions particular grounds for prescribing a higher-cost product. "If there's no specific reason, then we go for the best price we can get," Dr. Thomas says. When it comes to the highly advertised, high-cost products, such as Nexium for heartburn, Dr. Thomas talks to her cadre of pharmacists about using something like Prilosec instead, which provides about the same results and is now sold over-the-counter at a fraction of Nexium's price.

## Do You Need a Prescription Drug?

Sometimes you may not need a prescription drug. Dozens of over-the-counter products are available to you if your complaint is minor but still uncomfortable. While your pharmacist is not interested in trying to play doctor, he or she can help you save time and money by suggesting remedies that don't require a prescription.

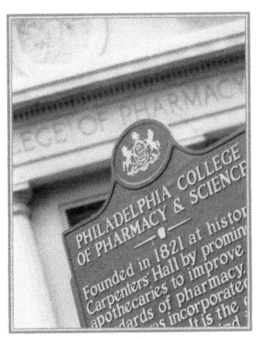

The Philadelphia College of Pharmacy
Photo courtesy of the college

"Try a pharmacist first, before going to a physician for some nonthreatening condition," suggests Daniel A. Hussar, Ph.D., Remington Professor of Pharmacy at the Philadelphia College of Pharmacy. He cites a case where a man in his sixties was experiencing some common cold symptoms. This sneezing, sniffling, coughing patient went to his pharmacy to find a product that would provide some relief. But he was bewildered by the array of products for every kind of cold and flu symptom.

Here's where a pharmacist can help. The man didn't need an analgesic for headaches, nor did he need an antihistamine for allergies he didn't have. When the man described his symptoms, how long he had been suffering, and some of the other drugs he was taking, the pharmacist was able to determine a specific product to fit the patient's needs—one without other chemicals that might only make things worse. In this kind of situation, a savvy pharmacist can act as a self-medication advisor, saving you considerable time and money.

## PHARMACIST CARE MANAGERS

The role of pharmacist continues to evolve as the health-care system grows in size and complexity. Pharmacists are coming out from behind the counter to play much more of a role in patients' care management.

According to the American Pharmacists Association, many pharmacies have even set up private consulting areas and are beginning to make house calls. Some pharmacists are providing easy access medical monitoring services, such as "point-of-care" home diagnostic testing. Working with patients' physicians, these new wave pharmacies are helping patients get more control over their diseases. Some pharmacies are becoming miniclinics, handling some medical testing services on the premises, such as:

- Cholesterol screening and drug management
- Blood pressure screening and management
- Liver function testing for medications that require monitoring
- Kidney function testing
- Diabetes blood sugar monitoring and education
- Asthma education and monitoring
- Peripheral artery disease monitoring to test for artery narrowing or blockage
- Ulcer testing and treatment
- Anticoagulation monitoring for people on warfarin medication

The Ukrop Supermarket Pharmacy, which has about twenty outlets in and around Richmond, Virginia, has set up its own, in-house wellness centers that offer immunization shots, blood pressure checkups, cholesterol monitoring, bone-density screening for osteoporosis, and blood sugar testing for diabetes. Other testing devices and operations are in the works.

This pharmacy "clinic" trend is in its early stages and will take a while to spread nationwide. Some pharmacies are offering seminars where patients can hear physicians, pharmacists, nurses, dietitians, nutritionists, and other specialists

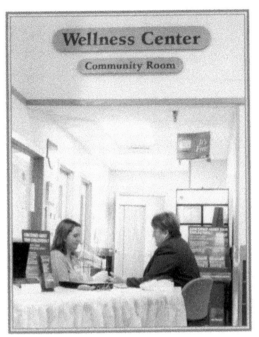

*A patient receives consultation at the Ukrop's Wellness Center in Richmond, Virginia.*
Photo courtesy of Ukrop's

talk about a wide variety of health problems.

Meanwhile you can usually get one-on-one help from your pharmacist on how to manage your medications to get the most benefit and play it safe. For example, has your doctor prescribed an inhaler to provide chest-wheezing allergy relief? Many people don't understand how to use an inhaler properly, which can lead to a real medical emergency. Your pharmacist can give you hands-on instructions in just a minute or two. Here's how it goes: You shake the inhaler vigorously, put it in your mouth, and inhale as you press the spray plunger. It's not as easy as it sounds!

Now that you've "met" your pharmacist and the pharmacy team, you're ready to select *your* pharmacy and develop a close, two-way relationship with your pharmacist-partner in self-care. In the next chapter, you'll see some of the ways you can benefit from this important relationship.

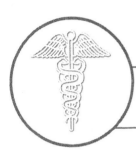

NINE

# Take Your Pharmacist to Lunch

In the previous chapter, you learned much more about the role pharmacists can and should play in medical care. You also discovered the depth and breadth of their training, and why these trained professionals are often under-used resources.

It's important to see your professional pharmacists as individuals, not as a mass of faceless pill pushers in white coats. Developing a relationship with your local pharmacy and the people who work there has real value, and not just of the dollars-and-cents kind. This chapter explains how you can work with your pharmacist and pharmacy staff to ensure the best possible medical support for your needs and at all times of your life.

## Choosing a Pharmacy and Pharmacist

The first thing to do is select a pharmacy that will become your base of operations for medicine management. It may be a chain drugstore, a pharmacy located in a medical clinic (the group with which your doctor is associated may have a pharmacy on its site), or an independent pharmacy.

How should you choose a pharmacy? For most of us, a convenient location is a valid reason for selecting a pharmacy, but it should not be the only one. Other factors may turn out to be more important, especially if you have several choices all in the same general vicinity.

When you walk into the store, does it look well stocked and clean? Are enough people working there so you won't have to wander up and down aisles looking for what you need? Does the pharmacy offer all the medicine consulting services you need? Is the pharmacy open during hours that you will find convenient? And does the pharmacy stay open as long as the rest of the store, or are its hours shorter? It's good to find this out.

If at all possible, find a pharmacy that makes you feel comfortable, as if you are a valued customer; you want to feel in charge of your own care. Remember, you're trying to stay healthy by managing your medicines properly. Their business is supplying the medicines and information you need, as well as the kind of service to keep you coming back.

"The selection of a pharmacy and a pharmacist is as important as selecting a physician," says Dr. Hussar of the Philadelphia College of Pharmacy. "Unfortunately," Dr. Hussar says, "some pharmacies are so busy and understaffed nobody has time to interact with patients to provide the information they need." If this is the case at your neighborhood pharmacy, don't let the convenience overshadow other concerns. Instead, keep shopping around to find a pharmacy where you can do business in a less hectic atmosphere—a place where you can build a relationship that focuses on you, the patient, working closely with your physician and a well-trained pharmacist. Sometimes independent pharmacies try to provide more individualized attention to compete with national chains.

A quick note: Even when you get to know a person behind the counter as your "personal" pharmacist, you should become familiar with other staffers who work there. If your pharmacist is unavailable one day, having a friendly "backup" pharmacist or technician with whom you feel comfortable will allow you to get the help you need when you need it.

Do you know the names of some of the pharmacists who hand over your medications and have you sign receipts? Starting right now, you should make it your business to get to know the health-care specialists you are dealing with. You don't have to wait until you have a prescription in hand. Even if you're just picking up a bottle of Tums to keep on your night table, why not take the time to stop by the pharmacist counter? (Of course, if it's very crowded, ask a staff person when might be a good time to stop back and ask some questions. Most pharmacies have slower and busier times, so aim for a first chat when it's quiet. That way, your pharmacist can give you more complete attention.)

Begin by explaining that you are a customer who would appreciate the help of a professional to ensure you're taking medicines wisely. You may want to mention what coverage you do or don't have, adding that you're also interested in trying to keep down the cost of medication. Add that you're concerned about drug interactions and you're hoping that working with your pharmacist will make it safer for you to take whatever your doctor prescribes. Ask if you can make an appointment to bring in the contents of your medicine chest to discuss with the pharmacist. (This is called "brown bagging," and in chapter 10 you'll learn how it works.)

## IS THERE REALLY LUNCH INVOLVED?

Although this chapter is called "Take Your Pharmacist to Lunch," most people will not share a meal with a local pharmacist. However, some customers actually do take their pharmacist to lunch or, at least, for a cup of coffee or a soda nearby as a friendly, get-to-know-you gesture.

Remember that any given pharmacy has literally thousands of prescription and nonprescription drugs. You can't possibly know how to sift through all the combinations of products that might be dangerous if mixed with drugs you have at home. To sum up, a pharmacist can become your guide, your professional consultant, and your purchasing agent to steer you through this medicinal and economic maze.

If it's at all possible, select a pharmacy and stick with it. Bouncing around from one pharmacy to another spreads out your medicine records and you have less of a chance to get to know a pharmacist for easier consultation. And if you don't concentrate on one location, pharmacists may not know your complete medication history. By focusing on one location, your pharmacist can record, and keep updating, your computer-generated personal medication profile, which includes all your prescribed medicines from various physicians, plus all the over-the-counter items you take either regularly or on occasion.

Suggestion: When you travel, take a printout of your personal profile medicine records to show to an out-of-town doctor or pharmacist if needed. This is especially important if you happen to end up in a hospital emergency room. It will be safer if the emergency room personnel know what medicines you are taking.

## Geriatric Red Flags

As you age your body chemistry changes, which can make some medicines dangerous. For example, amitriptyline (brand name Elavil, made by Merck) is prescribed for patients with depression who have difficulty sleeping. According to the American Society of Consultant Pharmacists, whose members work in facilities for the elderly, this drug can cause a Parkinson's-like shuffling gait that, in turn, can cause loss of balance and dangerous falling episodes. Pharmacists can suggest other drugs that work without this potential danger. You can get a list of drugs that might be dangerous for seniors and a directory of pharmacists (by state and city) who have been specially trained in geriatric medicine. For more information, go to www.seniorcarepharmacist.com.

## TAKING INVENTORY

Once you have established a relationship with a pharmacy, where you are known and respected as a good customer, the next step is to round up all your pill bottles, including prescription and nonprescription medicines, herbal products, vitamins, whatever. Make an appointment to bring all this stuff into your pharmacy for analysis (this is explained in the next chapter). Some pharmacies may charge a modest fee for this medication analysis, but it is well worth it. Remember, the older you are, the more physicians you see, and the more medicines you take, the more you need the advice and counsel of a pharmacist.

## PHARMACISTS WHO SAVED THE DAY

The average pharmacy encounter is brief, and for most customers may be cordial but not substantial. However, many pharmacists consider each encounter with a customer an opportunity to check up on a person's condition and find out if he or she is experiencing any related problems.

## Important Questions to Ask Your Physician or Pharmacist

It's a good idea to take a pad and pencil with you when you visit your doctor's office. Before you go in, you should jot down details of symptoms you are experiencing (such as upset stomach, dry cough, insomnia, blurred vision, or difficulty swallowing food). Jot down any other peculiarities, such as the fact that you have discovered a small lump on your neck or elsewhere on your body. Your notepad can also be used to record suggestions your doctor might make regarding your lifestyle, such as diet and exercise regimens. With your notepad handy, it's a good idea to ask questions about any medication that is being prescribed.

At the pharmacy, you'll also need your notepad when you pick up your prescription. Even if your medicine comes with a printed insert, you should feel free to ask for direct help in taking it correctly. (Besides, the print is often a bit small.)

Here are some of the most important questions you can ask:

1. What is the name of this medication?

2. What is it supposed to do for me?

3. How does the medicine work?

4. How will I know if it's working? (Will the doctor do a follow-up test?)

5. What time of day should I take it? (Before, after, with meals? Every four hours?)

6. What is the exact dose I am supposed to take? How often do I take that?

7. Are there any special instructions about how to take this medication? (For instance, if I have trouble swallowing the pill, can I crush it and mix it in juice?)

8. Should I be concerned about how this medicine will interact with my other prescription medicines? What about over-the-counter drugs?

9. Will this medication interact with any foods I may eat?

10. Am I allowed to drink alcohol while I am on this medication?

11. For how long should I continue to take this medication?

12. What should I do if I miss a dose (or forget to take it)?

13. Where and how should I store this medicine? (Bathroom, refrigerator, night table?)

14. If I experience side effects, should I call the doctor's office? Which side effects are important enough to call about, and which are not?

15. Can I renew this prescription? How many times?

16. If I don't use all the medicine in the bottle, should I keep it for later? Will it lose strength over time? Should I discard any pills I don't take?

17. Is there a generic version of this medicine? If there isn't now, do you think there will be soon?

18. Is there any activity I shouldn't do while I am taking this medicine? (Drive, sit in the sun, travel outside the United States?)

19. If I become ill and vomit the pill up after swallowing it, what should I do? (Take another? Call the doctor?)

20. Is this medication available in chewable form? (If not, for children can it be hidden in food, crushed in milk or juice, or otherwise "sneaked" in?)

Don't be embarrassed about asking questions—your good health depends on it. People who don't speak up are more likely to accidentally overdose or diminish the potency of their medicine by taking or storing it incorrectly.

Sometimes an attentive pharmacist can intervene in a way that makes a tremendous difference. Here are three examples.

## SAVING MONEY

Richard, a retired salesman in his seventies who lives in Asheville, North Carolina, came to the Kerr Drug pharmacy counter with a prescription for a refill of Prilosec, a drug he'd been taking to calm his indigestion, reduce his heartburn, and lessen the effects of acid reflux disease. At the time, Richard learned that the cost of this prescription was more than $100 for a month's supply—almost $3.50 a pill. He told pharmacist Beth D. Greck that he didn't know how he would manage. Each month, he had little money left after paying his rent and other fixed expenses. After talking with Richard's physician, Greck suggested he switch to

Pepcid AC, a much less expensive, over-the-counter remedy that has the same ingredients as the popular prescription drug. "It worked like a charm," Richard said when he came in to thank the pharmacist, "and it didn't cost me a lot of money." And Richard now has a pharmacist friend to consult about other medical concerns when he needs one.

## HELPING MAKE A DIAGNOSIS

Margaret, a widow in her fifties who also lives in Asheville, North Carolina, took advantage of her Kerr Drug pharmacy's new screening service aimed at detecting diabetes. Pharmacist Beth Greck reports that the woman's blood sugar count was very high, more than 200, and referred her immediately to her physician. Undetected diabetes can cause real damage to the body, and this brief test helped a customer avoid developing serious, long-term medical complications, Margaret sent a note to the pharmacy, praising the pharmacists for offering a ser-vice that may have saved her life.

## AVOIDING PRESCRIPTION DISASTER

Brian Jensen, a pharmacist with the Lakeshore Apothacare, Inc. in Two Rivers, Wisconsin, had a fifty-eight-year-old customer named Robert on renal dialysis for kidney disease. Jensen says that Robert's physician's office phoned in a prescription for 500 milligrams of ciproflaxin, a drug intended to quickly heal an ulcer on Robert's foot. Jensen noticed that the prescription said to take the medicine four times a day for two weeks, and figured something was wrong.

After phoning the physician's office, the pharmacist learned that his instincts were correct. Robert was supposed to take his medicine only once a day, not four times. "Four doses a day could have caused central nervous system problems," Jensen says.

How could this have happened? The code for taking a medicine once a day is "Q.D." while the code to take medicine four times a day is "QID." In this case, a hastily written period between the Q and the D can make it look like QID. Robert says he "thanks the pharmacy people again and again" every time he comes in.

# TAKING CHARGE OF YOUR SAFETY

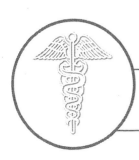

TEN

# EXAMINE YOUR
# CHEMICAL MIX

Y ou may think of your medicine cabinet as a fairly friendly place. Aside from personal hygiene items, such as toothpaste, shaving gear, mouthwash, and the like, you've probably got some popular painkillers, plus the usual cough and cold remedies, not to mention several prescription drugs. And, the older you get, say, sixty and above, the more likely you will be seeing three or more prescription labels lined up in there.

Friendly as it may look, your medicine cabinet can be a dangerous place where you might easily take out a mixture of drugs that could do some real harm. Pharmacist Mark Boesen, who warned about bad drug mixtures with herbal and other supplements in chapter 6, says, "There are so many different chemicals in those medicine cabinet bottles, you can't assume that any one of them, prescribed or over-the-counter, is absolutely safe when mixed in with other medications you are taking."

The people most at risk are those who are seeing several physicians, all of whom are writing prescriptions, possibly without knowing about all the other medications you are taking. Your physicians may know about some of your prescription drugs but not all of them.

They also may not know about the over-the-counter remedies you are taking, either because you forgot to mention them or because you didn't think they were worth mentioning. These seemingly innocuous nonprescription remedies can become a source of danger if combined with prescription drugs or other nonprescription medicines.

"Unfortunately, we don't have a universal patient record system, and this means other medical people who are treating you may not know about all the drugs you are taking," says Allen J. Vaida, Pharm.D., executive director of the Institute for Safe Medication Practices in Huntingdon Valley, Pennsylvania. He suggests making a written list of all your health-care professionals and adds that the list should include such people as dentists, optometrists, podiatrists, and nurses—everyone and anyone who is authorized to prescribe painkillers, antibiotics, sedatives, or blood pressure drugs.

For example, dentists are likely to prescribe pain medications when they have to do some drilling and gum work. They may also prescribe a tranquilizer if a patient appears to be overly anxious, or antibiotics to prevent an infection. It all goes into what we call "your chemical mix."

## PLAYING DOCTOR

All too many patients prescribe their own regimen of drugs, using guesswork, hearsay, and the odd magazine or newspaper article, without any real medical knowledge. Many of these patients end up taking drugs that are outdated, unsuitable, or truly unsafe.

"Some misguided patients may have leftover drugs in their medicine cabinets and use them inappropriately later on," says John R. Horn, Pharm.D., professor of pharmacy at the University of Washington School of Pharmacy in Seattle. "These 'medicine hoarders' think they're saving money by keeping the drugs they didn't finish." Then when they contract an ailment they believe shows similar symptoms, they resort to the old standbys in the medicine cabinet. "They may feel pain or discomfort and take one of the old drugs," Dr. Horn says, "not realizing that now they are also taking some new drug that could produce a dangerous chemical mixture."

He gives the example of a woman in her sixties who was involved in a severe automobile accident. At first police thought she might have been drinking or on some illicit drugs. Upon further investigation, they learned that she had been taking the tranquilizer Valium for anxiety and then on top of it swallowed some leftover Tylenol Number 4 (which is Tylenol plus codeine) for her back pain.

This ill-advised combination caused her to become woozy and doze off at the wheel. By self-medicating for pain, she inadvertently doubled up the sedative effect of the codeine to a perilous level.

Another example of a bad chemical mix is the following hypothetical scenario: A seventy-nine-year-old man having trouble sleeping is prescribed a relatively mild sedative by his physician. Later in the week the man goes to his dentist for root canal work and is given a tranquilizer and a painkiller. According to David Knapp, Ph.D., dean of the University of Maryland School of Pharmacy, when added together, these drugs are powerful enough to make the patient in this scenario feel dizzy and off balance. The overdrugged patient could easily fall and fracture his hip. Dr. Knapp says this kind of drug-induced accident is rarely reported in medical literature anymore because it is so common. Not only that, but because the admitting diagnosis in the hospital was listed as a fractured hip and not a drug interaction, the frequency of such events is probably underestimated.

## SOME WAYS THAT PATIENTS FAIL AT SELF-CARE

One of the most frequent problems reported by physicians and pharmacists arises when a patient is prescribed an antibiotic medication that is supposed to be taken for fourteen days to destroy the bacteria that caused the infection. But after a week the patient suddenly feels a lot better and stops taking the drug. When another infection comes up many months later, the patient starts popping the rest of the antibiotic pills on the theory that if it worked well before, it might again. But using old antibiotics, which should have been completed the first time around, can lead to a serious complication. The bacteria in your system may build up a resistance to a whole range of drugs, which will likely make curing some future infection much more difficult. Many of these infections not only develop a resistance to the medicine, they come back much stronger at a future date.

Another problem may exist: That old antibiotic might not work at all on the new infection because different microorganisms may be involved. By taking the wrong antibiotic without a doctor's supervision, you may end up losing time, money, and your good health.

And beware of family members or friends who want to play doctor! They may sound sure that they have just the right thing for your cough, cold, pain, or whatever. But Brian J. Isetts, Ph.D., associate professor of pharmacy at the University of Minnesota College of Pharmacy, says, "More than 10 percent of drug therapy problems involve medications that patients obtain from friends or family."

Dr. Isetts tells about a fifty-three-year-old man who had never before experienced a negative reaction to a penicillin derivative. When he came down with a bad cold, a friend passed along a bottle of penicillin pills that had been sitting in his medicine cabinet for more than three years. The friend should have finished all the pills himself or thrown them away. But choosing what seemed to be thriftiness over good sense, he saved the medicine for possible future use.

It was a bad decision.

The man with the cold not only didn't get better, he came down with a severe case of hives, and had to be rushed to the nearest hospital emergency room for treatment. A chemical evaluation of the old penicillin the man had taken suggested that the medicine's chemicals may have been degraded to a point where they could have triggered the severe allergic reaction.

Pharmacists and physicians warn to never use outdated prescriptions, leftover medications (it's best to flush it down the toilet), or over-the-counter medications past their expiration date. And never take someone else's prescribed medication.

## RISKY MIXES

There's a reason pharmacists have to spend years in classes learning which drugs can be safely mixed and which ones may present dangers to patients. The average

---

### Warning!

Don't Use These Drugs:

- Outdated prescriptions
- Leftover pills
- Rx gifts from family or friends

---

well-educated, well-read individual doesn't know enough to mix even a few drugs with complete safety.

Some chemicals in commonly used prescription and nonprescription drugs can create havoc when mixed with other drugs. Drug names that end in "ofen," for example, should be handled with considerable care. Ibuprofen is found in pain remedies such as Advil and Motrin. Related chemicals occur in Aleve and Naproxyn. Orudis KT has ketoprofen, which has a related ingredient.

Another widely used (and "ofen"-sounding) drug is acetaminophen, which can be found in more than four hundred prescription and nonprescription drugs. You may be taking Tylenol, a popular over-the-counter product with acetaminophen as its main ingredient. You may also be taking a drug for headaches, and another for arthritis, and yet still another for your coughs and colds. They all may contain acetaminophen, which can be found in a variety of over-the-counter products for pain, coughs, colds, and fever. It is shockingly easy to overdose with acetaminophen. This is why consumers should always read drug labels or package inserts with care. When you look for medications with "ofen" or "ophen" at the end, you may be surprised to discover how many contain the same or similar ingredients. It's worth taking a few minutes to ask a pharmacist about the product you are buying. Does it clash with other drugs or food products? Will it hurt you if taken along with other drugs? *You need to know.*

Be extra careful when you're taking antibiotics. They may contain an ingredient that interacts dangerously with medicine you're already counting on. One woman in her late thirties who was taking birth control pills got a shock when her doctor told her that she was pregnant. The newly pregnant patient had been taking amoxicillin, an antibiotic, which can decrease the effectiveness of birth control medications.

The don't-mix list gets longer and longer. Some examples:

**Wellbutrin and Zyban.** A man in his sixties was taking a prescribed drug, Wellbutrin, for depression. He also started using Zyban to help him stop smoking. A single chemical, buproprion, was the main ingredient in both drugs. The patient was also taking another antidepressant. The triple dose made the man feel so nauseated and sleepy that he was unable to get out of bed in the morning.

**Digoxin and Tagamet.** A woman in her seventies was taking digoxin, a generic drug for atrial fibrillation, a fairly common heart-rhythm problem. Without speaking to any of her health-care team, she walked into a pharmacy and purchased Tagamet, a popular heartburn remedy. Unfortunately, the chemicals in Tagamet interfered with the digoxin. The result: a serious heart incident that required emergency transportation to a nearby hospital emergency room.

**Depression meds and ibuprofen.** People who are taking prescribed drugs for depression as well as an anti-inflammatory painkiller with ibuprofen, according to University of Washington pharmacy professor John Horn, "increase the risk of gastrointestinal bleeding by more than fifteen times."

**Aspirin and ibuprofen.** People taking a daily aspirin, even the low-dose ones for the prevention of clogged arteries, should know that painkillers with ibuprofen as the main ingredient can interfere with the aspirin's therapeutic effect. In this case, you should check with your pharmacist about trying another painkiller that won't interfere with your daily aspirin dosage.

**Blood pressure meds and ibuprofen.** People who suffer from high blood pressure should be extra wary of painkillers with ibuprofen. According to Dr. Isetts, "the ibuprofen family chemicals constrict renal (kidney) arteries, which further elevates the blood pressure." This is especially important for people who suffer from chronic pain, such as arthritis, and are taking ibuprofen derivatives regularly.

## ORGANIZED DRUG MONITORING

Because drug interactions can harm you in many ways, you need to set up a system that allows you to keep track of everything you are ingesting, including prescription drugs, nonprescription drugs, herbal remedies, and even some food and drink products.

The first step is taking an inventory. Possibly the best way to do this—and a way to keep your list up-to-date and in professional hands—is to start by putting everything in your medicine cabinet and perhaps some items from your kitchen cabinet into a big brown paper bag (or any other bag that is strong and holds a lot).

This is unofficially called "brown bagging" in the pharmacy trade. Here's how it

## Morning Warning

Do you like grapefruit juice with your coffee for breakfast in the morning? If so, you should know that chemicals in grapefruit called bioflavonoids can interact negatively with various drugs, including anti-depressants, cholesterol control medicines (statins), and drugs that control blood pressure. Some drugs, such as the antibiotic ciproflaxin (trade name Cipro) can interfere with the body's ability to get rid of caffeine, which in turn can keep you awake—which might cause you to reach for a sleep aid.

A Virginia woman in her late fifties was taking an expensive "statin" drug to bring down her elevated cholesterol level. But no one ever told her to stop drinking a large glass of grapefruit juice for breakfast each day. The natural chemical in the juice interfered with the body's normal mechanism to metabolize the statin, and it accumulated in her system. Her physician became suspicious when she complained about extreme muscle weakness. When he asked her about her diet, he discovered the grapefruit juice problem. Prescription: no more grapefruit juice. Outcome: the statin level in her blood came down, the muscle problem disappeared, and her cholesterol is normal.

works. Talk with some pharmacies in your area to see if they are willing to set up a drug monitoring system for you. Most pharmacies will be glad to cooperate—not only to help you avoid medication interactions, but because it means you will become a regular customer and will tell others about the wonderful service you are getting. Some pharmacies are even setting up patient-information seminars that show how brown bagging works initially and as part of a continuing effort to monitor your drug intake.

Once your "patient profile" is set up on the pharmacy computer, all your medications can be checked out and entered. If you have used the pharmacy before, some of this information may already be on file. Now you will be adding drugs you've obtained from other pharmacies and anything else you may have purchased on-line. (If you've begun to use an on-line pharmacy, you should talk to a pharmacist on the phone and set up a patient profile there as well.) The trick is to keep all your drug outlets informed about what you're taking.

Always keep your pharmacy resources up to date. It might seem like a bother, but it can help both prevent risky drug interactions and, at the same time, save you money. Aside from the prescription drugs, over-the-counter products, and supplements you are taking, you might want to show your pharmacist a weeklong food journal so you can begin a dialogue about food and drink products that might affect your health. These may include broccoli, leafy vegetables, grapefruit juice, coffee, alcohol, and many more. The pharmacist may suggest other options to replace foods that interfere with your medications.

You may also want to set up a contact sheet listing the physicians you see regularly and provide a copy to your brown-bag pharmacy headquarters so they can stay in touch. Ask your physician's office staff if they can help set things up. Let everyone know that to ensure the best possible care, you would appreciate their help in making certain all your medications are well documented and on file.

Ask your physicians and your pharmacist if they have regular access to drug interaction information on-line or through a constantly updated, loose-leaf file. Some physicians might not have complete drug interaction information available and up-to-date, but pharmacists are required by law to have it available. They need to make sure every new drug that comes along can be cross-referenced to other products that might interact poorly.

## PRINTOUT PROTECTION

Once you've set up a system to help you monitor all the drugs and related products you are taking, you'll need to get printouts from your pharmacy (or pharmacies, if you work with more than one) to take with you when you visit any new health-care professional who might be writing prescriptions for you.

The more details your profile contains, the more valuable your printouts become. These should include any allergies; any significant changes in your blood pressure in the past year; and any adverse reactions you've had to drug products, either prescribed or over-the-counter.

But a patient-profile printout needs to be continuously attended to. You should keep several updated printouts on file at your home and at your workplace. When you visit a new physician or a new pharmacy (including on-line pharmacies) present your printout or fax it to the attending pharmacist for reference.

A final note: When you travel, tuck an updated patient profile in your carry-on bag or your briefcase. If anything happens while you're away from home, your records will be a ready reference. That way you lessen the chances of being given any medication that could put you at risk or interact badly with medication you're already taking. Savvy international travelers do this. It's time that you did too.

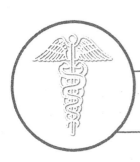

# ELEVEN

# TAKING MEDICINES CORRECTLY

Getting the drugs you require is vital; making sure that you're not taking anything that will interact badly with another of your medications is equally important. But perhaps the most critical job you have as a smart patient and drug consumer is ensuring that you're taking your medicine *right*.

Beverly is a fifty-year-old teacher who visited her physician complaining of stress, nervousness, and swollen ankles. Her physician took a careful history, which included several checks of her blood pressure. Beverly's blood pressure was 170 over 100, which is considered seriously, even dangerously, high. Her physician advised her to speak with a counselor about the emotional stress she was experiencing and prescribed a diuretic to flush water from her body's tissues, which in turn should help lower her blood pressure and reduce the swelling in her legs.

Her physician gave Beverly a prescription for hydrochlorothiazide in 25-milligram tablets. The instructions on the pill bottle simply said, "Take 1 tablet every day." Simple enough, Beverly thought. She took the bag from the pharmacist, set the bottle on the counter in her kitchen, and the following morning took her first pill. Because Beverly rarely eats breakfast, she took the pill with just a sip of water and headed off to school. At lunch she complained to a friend of an upset stomach, and she also noticed that she felt lightheaded throughout the day. When she got home, it was too late to call the doctor, but as she picked up the pill bottle, wondering if its label contained any advice or information, she noticed the bag still sitting on the counter. Inside the bag, she discovered a sheet of patient prescription information she hadn't noticed before. She rarely took any medicine, and she hadn't known to look for it. (The pharmacist hadn't mentioned it to her, either.)

## THE INFORMATION SHEET

The info sheet explained that her pill, a generic prescription diuretic, should be taken in the morning with food or milk to reduce stomach upset. Ah, she thought, that was her first mistake, but at least now she knew. She read further down, discovering a lengthy list of potential side effects, including lightheadedness or dizzy spells. That explained what she'd experienced during the day.

She was amazed to discover under "Precautions" that people taking hydrochlorothiazide should avoid prolonged sun exposure and wear protective clothing when they were outdoors. She also learned that she might experience blurry vision, loss of appetite, itching, headache, or weakness as her body adjusted to the diuretic.

The page also offered advice about potential drug interactions. Beverly found it a little unnerving to learn that she shouldn't take a decongestant while taking this drug because it might increase her heart rate and counteract her blood pressure medicine. The instructions recommended she inform her physician if she was taking ibuprofen, a common over-the-counter medication for aches and pains. She rarely took any medicine for a headache, and when she did it was usually Tylenol (acetaminophen), which wasn't on the warning list, and she wondered why. She decided to discuss it with her CVS pharmacist.

The information sheet was remarkably thorough, she thought. It mentioned that taking this drug might reduce the level of potassium in her blood and suggested consulting her physician about increasing her dietary potassium. Beverly recalled that bananas were high in potassium, and she resolved to begin bringing them to school with her lunch.

The last section described the safe way to store her prescription—at room temperature and away from moisture and sunlight. She usually kept medications in her bathroom medicine chest, but this info sheet said, "Do not store in the bathroom." How often, she wondered, had she made such mistakes when taking a prescribed drug? She might have continued to do everything wrong if she hadn't spotted the paper in the store bag. What if she'd thrown it out without finding it? And how many other people did the same thing?

Sadly, too many people don't understand the right way to take a particular medication, even when they receive the accompanying information sheet with each prescription. Some find the print too small or the language too confusing. Others glance at it but ignore important points (like where to store your pills so they don't lose potency). Still others can't keep the different instructions straight for each medicine they take.

Many seniors ingest a mix of medicines—some that they should take with food, and others on an empty stomach; some that can be taken with almost any liquid, and others that will lose strength if you happen to swallow them just before or just after you drink your morning grapefruit juice. Some pills are for just before bed, while others must be taken in the early morning. Some pills need to be taken several times a day, some every other day. Even a clear-headed and well-educated adult can easily feel overwhelmed.

## WHAT'S THE PROBLEM?

PhRMA, the Pharmaceutical Research and Manufacturers of America, posted on its Web site (www.phrma.org) the following list of common mistakes people make when taking medicine:

- They don't get their prescriptions filled, or they forget to refill.
- They underdose, taking less medicine than prescribed, taking it less often, or skipping doses.
- They stop the medicine too soon, whether or not symptoms disappear.
- They overdose, taking too much of a medicine or taking it too often.
- They mistime their doses, not taking them at the right intervals or times of day.

Do any of these sound familiar? Many people are "guilty" of at least one or more mistakes on this list, at least occasionally, and the results could be serious. Some medications are affected by a break in continuity, losing some of their effectiveness if a day or two are missed. Medications for some conditions, such as heart disease, high blood pressure, epilepsy, asthma, depression, and prevention of blood clots must *never* be stopped suddenly. Your body may experience withdrawal symptoms if you forget your medicine or don't take it for even a few days. Some medicines don't work properly if you don't take the whole dose.

Let's take a look at these prescription "goof ups."

### OUT OF MONEY

Did you decide not to fill a prescription because of financial hardship? Before you risk your health, consult the money-saving strategies in the next section of this book to decrease your costs. Sometimes a delay in taking a medicine can cause a serious problem.

### FORGETTING REFILLS

Did you forget to refill your prescription before you ran out, then find yourself without your necessary medication for a day or more? If you refill monthly, mark your calendar—make an appointment with yourself to ensure that you won't be without your pills. If you have had trouble in the past remembering when to take your medicine or when to get your refills, talk to your pharmacist. Many useful and inexpensive devices are available, including labeled pill boxes, reminder calendars, stickers, and special packaging that should make it easier.

### WORRIES ABOUT A FULL DOSE

Did you deliberately underdose yourself because of fears about the medication's strength or perhaps because of worrisome side effects you experienced earlier on a full dose? *Call your doctor immediately.* You don't have the knowledge to alter your prescription safely. You need medical advice to be certain you aren't putting yourself in any danger.

### THINK YOU'RE CURED

Did you stop taking your medicine for an infection once it appeared to be gone? Some bacteria develop a resistance to antibiotics if they're not fully wiped out by the entire course of treatment. If this happens too often, you could find yourself fighting another infection that doesn't respond to anything left on the antibiotic shelf. This is a real public health problem, so don't contribute to it by taking anything less than all the medicine your doctor advises.

### FORGETTING YOU TOOK IT

Did you overdose by forgetting you took your medicine and taking it twice? You may want to use one of those handy "count-it-out-in-advance" boxes with daily compartments for your pills, available at any drugstore. This makes it harder to overdose, because once you take the pills you've put into the daily compartment, you're done.

### MEASURING IT RIGHT

Liquid medication may require special instructions. According to the American Academy of Pediatrics, research shows that many people do not understand the right way to measure liquid medicines. For example, many use household teaspoons, which usually do not hold a true teaspoon of liquid. Special devices, such as marked oral syringes, make it easy to measure the right dose.

### ADJUSTING THE TIMING

Did you take your medicine at the wrong time because you overslept or were too tired to wait the correct interval before going to sleep? Talk to your physician about the problem, and consider setting a "medication alarm clock" if your prescription requires such an exacting schedule. If you're confused about the terminology of dosing, ask. For example, ask if "four doses daily" means taking a dose every six hours around the clock or just spaced during your regular waking hours.

## A NEW SYMPTOM MAY BE IMPORTANT

Sometimes even when you take your medicine exactly as your physician prescribes, you still experience an unexpected or disturbing new symptom. While some symptoms caused by a new medication may not be serious, if you develop a rash or shortness of breath while taking a medicine, especially an antibiotic, do *not* take the next dose until you have talked with your doctor.

The symptom may be caused by a food or drink interaction that wasn't listed on the bottle or package as a possible concern. Some foods or drinks can make your medicine work too fast or too slowly or even not at all. Others may cause a life-threatening reaction. Alcohol can be extremely dangerous when taken with some medicines.

Here are some combinations that have produced health problems in many consumers:

- MAO (monoamine oxidase) inhibitors (antidepressants) and aged or fermented foods (beer or red wine, most cheeses, sausage and processed meats, smoked fish, yogurt or sour cream)

- Tetracycline and milk products

- High blood pressure medicines and natural licorice

- Coumadin (a blood thinner) and liver or leafy green vegetables

## SAFETY BEGINS AT HOME—AND WITH YOU

It's important to keep safety precautions in mind when buying, using, and storing medicines. Make sure your children know about using medicine safely. Here are some valuable safety practices to keep in mind:

- When you buy medicine, check the package at the store to make sure that no one else has opened it. Tamperproof caps have made many products safer, but other problems can occur.

- Check to see if the medicine looks normal and just as you expected it to look. If you think it looks or smells odd or old, ask your pharmacist to check it.

- Never take anyone else's prescription medicine, and flush any unused medicine down the toilet.

- Keep your medicine in its original container so you don't forget what the drug is or what it's for.

- Keep all medications out of reach of children—locked up if possible. People who infrequently have young visitors may not be prepared for small, inquisitive guests. If a child is using your bathroom, make certain every pill bottle is out of reach or under lock and key.

- Post the number of the Regional Poison Control Center next to your phone, and keep ipecac syrup (to induce vomiting) on hand for use *only if a poison specialist advises it.* Inducing vomiting is not always safe, so don't automatically reach for the ipecac.

- Teach children about medicine, and always call it "medicine," not "candy" or "drugs." Explain that medicine is only to help make them well if they are sick but when taken at any other time can be dangerous, like poison. You may also want to talk about the differences between prescription medicines and illegal drugs so that what's in your bedside pill bottles doesn't seem fascinating or encourage curiosity. And remember that "child-safety" caps are sometimes not childproof.

## What If You Can't Read Your Prescription Instructions?

Millions of Americans are rapidly approaching "the golden years" or already well over traditional retirement age. As the population ages, more and more products are being invented to ease the requirements of daily life. One of the more imaginative is the Talking Rx, marketed as "an innovative tool for taking prescriptions correctly." It may offer valuable help to anyone with visual impairment, especially someone who finds it hard to tell different medicines apart. If you have difficulty reading small print or tend to be a little forgetful, this product might be right for you. The elderly may need to have a friend, or someone else, record all the detailed information from their prescriptions, but once it's recorded, they're good to go.

Press a button, and a recorded voice tells you who this prescription is for, what it is called, and what it treats. It describes the pills by color; it tells you when and how to take them. It describes potential side effects and tells you to call your doctor if you experience any of them.

The Talking Rx fits on the bottom of your pill bottle, is water-resistant, operates on watch batteries, can record up to sixty seconds of information, and is reusable. Sold by the Millennium Compliance Company of Southington, Connecticut, it costs $15. For more information, go to www.talkingrx.com.

## A FEW MORE IMPORTANT GUIDELINES

You have your dose correct, you remember when to take it, and you never forget to get refills on time. You're well on your way to getting the most out of your medications, but here are more important points:

- Drink a few gulps of water to lubricate your esophagus before swallowing a pill. Also drink a glass of water *after* you have taken the medication.

- Shake well any liquid medication before you pour out a dose. Remember to use a medical measuring spoon, not a kitchen teaspoon.

- Keep drugs out of direct sunlight, humid places (such as the bathroom or near the kitchen sink), and hot automobiles. Don't store your drugs in the freezer or refrigerator unless instructed to do so.

- Don't stop taking a drug or change dosage without consulting your doctor.

- How some drugs affect you changes as you age, so ask your doctor about reviewing dosages of drugs you've been taking for a long time.

- Don't crush tablets or capsules. Many pills contain time-release medication that may work too fast if you crush the outside coating.

- Do not take or give medicine in the dark, without your glasses on, or while you are sleepy.

- Consult your doctor before taking any drug if you know or suspect you are pregnant or if you're breast-feeding.

- If you will be traveling, find out if your medication can be used in different climates.

You have valuable partners in your physician and your pharmacist, but ultimately safety begins with you!

# TAKING CONTROL
# OF YOUR MONEY

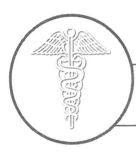

TWELVE

# BUYING RIGHT

Paying for prescriptions these days is a little tricky. The field breaks down into two categories: 1) Drugs that are covered by insurance plans and thus have little or no out-of-pocket expense in the form of a co-pay and 2) drugs that aren't covered and thus require a high out-of-pocket expense. No matter how large the co-pay, it is still a lot better than paying full price for a prescription.

Whether you have a prescription plan or not, the next step to saving money is to purchase a lower-cost generic drug instead of the more expensive brand name product—and to ask your physician about a less costly prescription medicine or even an over-the-counter remedy that has the same therapeutic effect. A good example can be found in the commercials aimed at allergy sufferers. Clarinex, made by the Schering pharmaceutical company, was getting all the TV commercial time. When this happened, you no longer heard about Claritin, the company's old standby.

Why? Because Claritin lost its patent protection and had to be sold against competition from other pharmaceutical companies. So the manufacturer came up with Clarinex, which was tweaked just enough to get a new patent and a much higher price tag. In addition, Claritin no longer requires a prescription and, after a brief stint as a generic drug, is now competing well in the over-the-counter marketplace.

In a sense, the manufacturer is enjoying the best of both worlds, having a high-priced prescription product and a low-priced mass-market product. Ask any pharmacist. Nine times out of ten, you'll be told that both products have pretty much the same therapeutic effect. If your doctor doesn't have a special reason for you to be taking Clarinex, why pay more?

## DOES IT MATTER WHERE YOU BUY?

What factors go into the price you pay at a local or chain pharmacy? They vary more than you might imagine. The first factor is usually business volume—as a rule, the big chains, such as Rite Aid, CVS, and Eckerd, have lower markups. They are willing to accept a smaller profit on individual items because they sell so much more than their smaller competitors.

Another factor is likely to be location—the cost of real estate where the store is located. High-volume operations can afford to be conveniently located, open longer hours, and perhaps offer more services than an independent.

But you may still decide you want to take your business to one of the smaller, independent pharmacies, which you often find in or near a medical building that houses physicians' offices. Are their markups higher? Usually, but there may be a trade-off. At an independent pharmacy, you may find the lines shorter and the service more personal—and more comprehensive. Ask yourself if it's worth paying a little more to get in and out quickly. The bottom line isn't just financial, then. The price you pay for your prescriptions is, at least in part, up to you.

## ARE PHARMACY MARKUPS FAIR?

The question is, are the prices you're being charged fair? Legal? People who find that they have to keep paying more for the same drug at their pharmacies may well believe that the pharmacies are charging more to increase their profit margins. Most pharmacists insist that this isn't so.

"It all starts with the manufacturing of the drug," says pharmacist Beth D. Greck. "That's where the biggest increases can be found."

Pharmacist Brian Jensen says, "We do not control the price; the insurers are really dictating prices for pharmacies because they present us with a contract that puts us in a take-it or leave-it situation." Jensen goes on to say that pharmacy profit margins on the prescription drugs they sell are no more than 2 to 3 percent. And the ultimate leveler, he says, is price comparison: "You can't hike your markups and be competitive with other stores in the area . . . Word gets around."

## LET THE BUYER BEWARE

Some pharmacies, however, apparently are price gouging—inflating the cost of generic and prescription drugs far above what the rest of the market is charging—according to an October 2003 ABC News.com report.

In Albuquerque, New Mexico, you could fill a prescription for the generic version of the heartburn drug, Pepcid, at Sam's Club for just $13, while the same prescription dispensed at a nearby pharmacy cost $87. These price differences came to light when the state attorney general sent interns to do random surveys of drugstores to check prices of some common prescriptions. One intern, Justin Woolf, said he purchased generic Prozac at one store for $15.72 while another store charged $54.99 for the same medicine.

WXYZ in Detroit also reported the same generic heartburn medicine selling at one store for $12 and another for $136. A Tampa, Florida, station reported a hypertension drug selling for $10.97 at one pharmacy and more than triple that price at another. And in Phoenix, KNXV found a generic antidepressant priced at $14 at one pharmacy and more than $267 at another.

It's up to you to decide if this is price gouging or simply "price variation," as one industry source described it, saying that some pharmacies boost prices on generic drugs because of the low profit margin on brand-new drugs. Whatever the reason, the range of prices is broad enough to suggest consumers must make a special effort to price their prescriptions at several local stores.

## FREE SAMPLES—A GIFT OR DISASTER WAITING TO HAPPEN?

Some physicians try to soften the financial blow of prescribing a pricey drug to a patient by providing plentiful free samples. But when it comes to patient safety, Jensen opposes the practice. Manufacturers' representatives provide drugs as a

## Have You Counted Your Pills Lately?

Another problem is that some pharmacies "underfill" the prescription when they run short on the medication, but bill insurance plans for the full amount. This practice, also called "short filling," costs the federal government millions because it occurs most often with Medicaid patients and others enrolled in federal health programs, according to the Associated Press.

Walgreens, the country's biggest pharmacy chain, was accused of short filling four million prescriptions and overcharging the government $21 million. It agreed to pay the government $7.6 million and adjust its computers to bill for partial prescriptions. This agreement settled claims in twenty-five states and Puerto Rico. Similar lawsuits were filed in Tennessee and Florida against Eckerd, claiming that it overcharged $11 million and short filled 180,000 prescriptions, but the Tennessee claim has been settled. According to court documents, both Walgreens and Eckerd denied any wrongdoing.

marketing tool, to encourage physicians to prescribe the company's new product. Patients are generally delighted, believing they are getting an expensive medication at no cost. But like so many free things, this gift comes with a drawback.

"The instructions that come with the sample may not always be clear," Jensen says, "and there is no pharmacist to question the patient about other drugs he or she may be taking—no chance to check out the patient's medication profile before the drug is consumed." He cites these serious mishaps:

- A physician phones in a prescription for Actonel, which is used to help prevent osteoporosis. The patient, a woman in her sixties, is questioned by the pharmacist when she picks it up. She had been taking 30-milligram samples daily before purchasing the drug—when in fact she should have been taking only one pill *a week*.

- A man in his forties was given a sample of an antibacterial eardrop that had to be used a couple of times a day to heal an infection. He ran out of the drops on a weekend when the physician wasn't available and had to stop the planned therapy. By stopping the drops before the infection was cured, the infection worsened so much that there was a real danger of hearing loss.

Jensen would like to see free vouchers or certificates given out by drug companies instead of the actual drug. This way, he says, the patient gets a free tryout but under much better supervision.

## COPING WITH CHANGING CO-PAYMENTS

If you have an insurance plan with prescription drug coverage, you may have faced a series of price hikes over the past year or so. You may have started out paying $5 as your share for a month's supply of a drug that costs $30, but then your co-pay increased to $10—and now it's up to $15. What's going on?

As the drug manufacturers continue to raise their prices, insurance plan managers say they have to keep increasing the co-pay for their members. Most companies or organizations will either scale back the overall medical coverage or increase the co-pay. People would generally rather pay more of a co-pay rather than have fewer benefits.

Members of AFTRA (American Federation of Television and Radio Artists), for instance, pay $3 or 25 percent of the discounted price for generics, whichever is greater. For a brand name, they pay $15 or 25 percent of the discounted price.

Group participants, of course, have to pay an insurance premium for the prescription drug coverage. At AFTRA this now runs around $250 a quarter—still a good deal if you have regular prescriptions to fill, because coverage includes care for your spouse.

With many plans you don't qualify for coverage until you reach a certain deductible amount. This deductible may include all of your medical costs, including prescription drugs, or it may not. It's worth taking the time to run the numbers just to see how much you are really paying for the coverage you're getting.

If you need assistance, ask if the staff in your physician's office can help sort things out. For seniors, it may be worthwhile to check with the local agency on aging for assistance referral. (Your local agency can usually be found in the Yellow Pages under "Aging Services" or "Senior Citizen's Service Organizations.") Your local information operator can also assist you in locating a city or county agency to help.

## HAS YOUR PLAN DROPPED YOUR MEDICINE?

Buying prescription drugs gets more and more complex, particularly as drugs travel along the continuum from hot brand name launch to eventual generic. You save some money when your drug goes generic, but many health insurance plans don't publicize a nasty little catch that occurs when your drug takes the last price step and goes over-the-counter. Once the product you rely on no longer needs a prescription, you won't get help paying for it. Most plans do not cover over-the-counter drugs, so you could end up paying more than you did when the drug needed a prescription. Review chapter 5, "Over-the-Counter Drugs," to see why some of these products might be used instead of those that require a prescription and vice versa. If your insurance plan doesn't cover an over-the-counter product that has a prescription equivalent, or near equivalent, you might find yourself in the unusual position of asking your physician for a prescription to replace your OTC product. Work the math. Which one saves the most money? Also, be sure to ask your doctor if there is any reason to choose one product over another.

## SHOULD YOU OPT OUT OF PRESCRIPTION DRUG COVERAGE?

While prescription drug benefits are a godsend for many people, paying for them may not be worth the cost. Consider how much you're paying for all your insurance premiums, what deductibles are required, and any co-pays. What are you paying for prescription drugs over a year? If you have no chronic illnesses and you're in general good health, your only medication costs during a year may be for a giant-size bottle of Tylenol and an occasional bottle of Tums.

But if you take medication for chronic illnesses such as arthritis or diabetes, if you catch strep throat from your school-age kids at least once a winter, if you suffer from more than infrequent skin problems or boils that require antibiotics, you very likely need prescription drug coverage.

Once you've added up what you spend over a year, divide the total by twelve to get a monthly average. Few people bother to figure out their actual monthly drug costs, but until you do, you may be overpaying for coverage you don't need or don't use.

If you're one of the lucky, healthy, infrequent prescription drug purchasers, consider a slightly revolutionary idea: *Insure yourself.* Why not fund your self-insurance plan through a special savings account set up especially for this purpose? Check with your tax advisor to see if you're eligible for a tax deduction or a credit for setting up such a medical savings account. If you don't have a tax advisor, you might be able to get some help from your bank, the regional Internal Revenue Service office, or the area agency on aging. Your telephone information operator can be of help with these numbers.

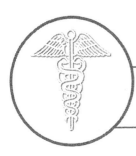

## THIRTEEN

## BUYING ONLINE

Whenever you open your online mailbox, you may find e-mail from strangers offering to sell you "generic Viagra" or some other drug. Do these marketers know something about you and is that why they've targeted you for this terrific offer? Absolutely not. These "spammers" are clogging the Internet daily with mass mailings, and many them are out to take your money and in many cases deliver a substandard product—or none at all.

Why are you and millions of others getting all this mail? Because selling prescription drugs online is a booming business, and everyone wants a piece of the action. According to the FDA, a huge surge in online purchasing has occurred over the past three years. It's quick, convenient, and you can place your order twenty-four hours a day and seven days a week. That's appealing to consumers who want the convenience of doing business and running errands on their schedule. Add to that the fact that you can often get a better price on your prescription by choosing an online pharmacy instead of heading for the corner drugstore.

But questions and concerns remain. Is it safe to do business with an online pharmacy? It's not the same as worrying whether your credit card transaction is secure. Prescription drugs are regulated substances that have the power to keep you healthy or make you very sick if they're tampered with or if you're sent the wrong dosage. Do you dare risk ordering your lifesaving prescription from UnknownDrugstore.com?

Some have compared the Internet to a type of Wild West, where consumer protection can be sketchy and e-mail addresses often little help in determining the source of a product, a company, or even a computer virus.

But the good news is that buying prescription drugs online can be a great way to compare prices, save money, and even get solid customer service. The key, as with any business transaction, is to know whom you're dealing with, what questions to ask, how to protect yourself, and how to be a confident and competent online consumer.

In this chapter you'll learn why it's definitely riskier to respond to a random e-mail drug offer than to order from Walgreens.com or CVS.com. You'll also discover how to choose among on-line suppliers and how buying online differs from shopping around your neighborhood.

## WHO'S SELLING DRUGS ONLINE?

The answer could be "just about anyone who wants to make a buck." Let's start with the simplest sources of online prescription drugs: the Internet stores of what are traditionally called "bricks-and-mortar" companies. In most towns and cities, you're likely to find chain drugstores such as CVS, Walgreens, Eckerd, and others. They operate in buildings—thus the bricks-and-mortar definition. In those stores you hand your prescription across the counter. You may have been chatting with the same pharmacist for years. You receive your pills right from the druggist's hands, and pay for them in the store with cash, a check, or your credit card.

Nearly all chain drugstores have opened online pharmacies, to earn part of the bonanza of online sales. Who purchases from these companies online? People just like you who are interested in saving money. People who like the convenience of shopping at midnight or 5 A.M. People who may be housebound or disabled and who prefer the ease of shopping without leaving their homes. Even computer buffs who like the idea of doing everything online.

But these companies are just one part of the online prescription drug equation. Who else wants to sell you Lipitor at a better price or even that frequently touted "generic Viagra"?

Drug dealers in countries all over the world now have access to American consumers through the Internet. Many of these are legitimate but may operate without the same regulations that protect U.S. citizens at home. Other sources, however, may have no connection with the medical profession, no trained personnel, and no safe medications to sell. It's up to you, the smart and savvy shopper, to decide where to take your business, and it's not always easy to know what you should do. In this chapter you'll find guidance to help you make the right decision.

## WORKING WITH AN ONLINE PHARMACY

What are the differences when ordering from an online pharmacy? Does anyone "out there" get to know you and treat you as an individual, not just a street address with a credit card?

Most on-line pharmacists you use regularly will maintain a "patient profile" that lists all the drugs you are taking. That's helpful, of course, but it only works if you keep the profile up to date and if you purchase all of your prescriptions from the same source. Some online pharmacies will send you an e-mail reminder when you're due for a refill. Others will alert you to significant price savings if and when your brand name drug goes generic or a generic drug you're taking goes "over-the-counter."

Most on-line pharmacies will mail your order to you at no additional cost. If you need a prescription quickly, you may have to pay a little extra for Priority or Express Mail. If you order from a drugstore chain, you may even be able to stop by the nearest outlet and pick up your prescription *without* having to stand in line. That's an appealing option to many prescription drug buyers who have spent valuable time waiting in a local drugstore.

But when you order online, you're not face to face with your pharmacist. You don't have the opportunity to bring in all the stuff from your medicine cabinet for review. Can you handle not speaking about your medicine with someone you know? The good news is that reliable on-line pharmacies all have certified pharmacists on duty around the clock, which can be an advantage over stores with regular hours. You can e-mail your questions and get a prompt answer. You can even get a pharmacist on the phone, as the legitimate online pharmacies have toll-free numbers.

Sounds wonderful, right? But all of this quick-service cost cutting does have a catch. You need to know that the source of your medication is dependable—and some businesses and individuals selling prescription drugs online are selling medicine that has been contaminated or diluted or is outdated and stale. "When you're on-line," warns Dr. Penna, "the other end of the line can be in some third-world country where anything goes."

## IS IT WORTH THE RISK?

With all the concerns about who's selling drugs on the Internet, is it really worth it to try and save money by purchasing online? The October 2003 *Consumer Reports* compared the cost of a "market basket" of five widely prescribed drugs (Celebrex, Lipitor, Norvasc, Prevacid, and Zoloft) when purchased online and when bought at major pharmacy chains, suppliers, and mass merchants. Look at the chart on page 147.

As you can see, it's possible to save as much as $100 by shopping around. Even if you buy your prescription drugs locally, you can save a few dollars (or more) by checking prices before you buy. Because prices may change often, it's worth checking back when it's time for a refill.

All of these online pharmacies are headquartered in the United States and are regulated by federal and state governments. More than seventy on-line pharmacies based in Canada have "reached out" to Americans who want to cut their drug costs. Canada also imposes strict regulations on its legitimate pharmacy outlets, so you can feel confident doing business with a Canadian pharmacy operating online.

The savings can be spectacular. Consider Eleanor, a fifty-seven-year-old American woman with chronic thyroid disease. She bought a ninety-day supply of a common thyroid medication called Synthroid from a Canadian pharmacy through www.affordableRx.com for *half* of what she usually paid at her neighborhood pharmacy.

But don't let the promise of big savings cloud your judgment. You have to be just as cautious when buying drugs online from Canada as with any online purchase. Some sources that list addresses in Canada are just using them as mail drops and are not regulated by the Canadian government. Their drugs could come from anywhere around the globe to be resold to unsuspecting customers who believe they are dealing with a trustworthy Canadian company.

## Price of "Market Basket" of Drugs

| Source | Price | Shipping cost |
|---|---|---|
| **ONLINE** | | |
| Familymeds.com | $377 | free |
| Costco.com | $395 | free |
| Drugstore.com | $398 | $1.49 |
| Eckerd.com | $408 | $1.95, free if order over $40 |
| Walgreens.com | $415 | $1.95 |
| Aarppharmacy.com | $420 | $2.25 |
| Clickpharmacy.com | $429 | $6.95, free if order over $65 |
| CVS.com | $454 | $1.95 |
| | | |
| **MASS MERCHANTS** | | |
| Costco | $399 | |
| Target | $421 | |
| Wal-Mart | $425 | |
| | | |
| **SUPERMARKETS** | | |
| Albertsons | $454 | |
| Safeway | $460 | |
| Kroger | $479 | |
| | | |
| **INDEPENDENTS** | (averaged $470) | |
| | | |
| **DRUG CHAINS** | | |
| CVS | $478 | |
| Eckerd | $481 | |
| Walgreens | $484 | |

Source: "Time to Switch Drugstores," Consumer Reports, October 2003.

When U.S. residents first began buying prescription drugs north of the border, the FDA told them to stop because it is technically illegal. As of this date, there is no evidence that any American who purchased drugs on-line from Canada has been arrested or warned by the FDA.

## How Can I Feel Safe Buying Drugs Online?

We've established that buying on-line can be convenient and can definitely save you money, but you have to know where your drugs are coming from. Does your online pharmacy have a working toll-free number, not just an answering service? Good. What about a real address, not a post office box? Good again. Here's another test: Did you use an online search engine or a recommendation from a friend or a reliable publication to find the online pharmacy? Or did you encounter a pitch for cut-rate drugs in an e-mail from someone you never heard of? Don't fall for a low-cost come-on that sounds like this: "Free Prescriptions for Weight Loss, Sexual Health, Muscle Pain, Pain Relief"—especially if the ad says in bold print "No Prescription Needed." Likewise, avoid such enticements as "Quick and Convenient Online Prescriptions. No prior prescription needed, no appointments, no waiting rooms."

Trying to save big bucks could mean buying big trouble. If the ad or e-mail doesn't list an address, *be warned*. If you just see an e-mail "order form," *don't bite*. These Web site outlaws may be offering super-cheap drugs, but the package you receive in the mail could be dangerously tainted.

Here's what happened to two people who purchased drugs online from prescription predators.

- A man in his fifties with a heart condition ordered Viagra from an online, no-address source. No prescription required, no physician checkup needed. After an evening of drinking, the man popped a Viagra, had sex with his girlfriend, and suffered a near-fatal heart attack. Had he seen his physician to request this prescription, he would have been warned that a man with his heart condition shouldn't use Viagra. Just because a drug is popular and provides a desirable outcome doesn't mean it is safe for everyone to take.

- A retired woman in her fifties needed an expensive, injectable medicine for her kidney condition. Barely able to make ends meet but afraid of what might happen if she didn't take the medication, she responded to an advertised online "pharmacy" that quoted rock-bottom prices. After she gave herself the first injection, her hip swelled up and she was rushed to the emergency room, where she almost died. It turned out that the bargain medicine in the self-injection tube contained water that was contaminated with bacteria.

## Drugs You Shouldn't Buy over the Internet

In December 2002 the FDA issued a consumer safety alert naming a group of drugs that should not be purchased on-line—because these medications have specific safety restrictions. The alert explains, "Also, drugs purchased from foreign Internet sources are not the FDA-approved versions of the drugs and are not subject to FDA-regulated manufacturing controls or FDA inspection of manufacturing facilities."

The drugs listed were:

**Accutane** (isotretinoin)

**Actiq** (fentanyl citrate)

**Clozaril** (clozapine)

**Lotronex** (alosetron hydrochloride)

**Mifeprex** (mifepristone or RU-486)

**Thalomid** (thalidomide)

**Tikosyn** (dofetilide)

**Tracleer** (bosentan)

**Trovan** (trovafloxacin mesylate or alatrofloxacin mesylate injection)

**Xyrem** (sodium oxybate)

The FDA warns that sophisticated technologies have made it fairly easy to produce potentially harmful counterfeit drugs. The agency has quadrupled its investigative force in an effort to stem the tide. During 2003 FDA investigators discovered more than two hundred thousand bottles of the cholesterol drug Lipitor that contained fake pills. According to the World Health Organization, up to 50 percent of the medicines sold in third-world countries are counterfeit. It's easy to understand why. When prices for any must-have product skyrocket, counterfeiters and organized crime move in, in search of an easy profit.

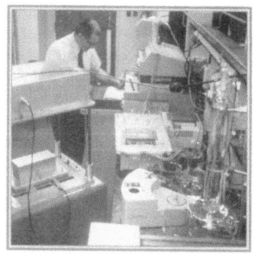

*Working in an FDA lab*
Photo courtesy of the Food and Drug Administration

## CALLING IN THE WATCHDOGS

Who's keeping us safe? The FDA is primarily concerned with the manufacture and sale of counterfeit drugs because of their potentially dangerous contents. But various state boards of pharmacy have the responsibility for regulating on-line pharmacies. Here's how the National Association of Boards of Pharmacy describes its role: "States protect their citizens by licensing out-of-state pharmacies that ship medications to patients in their jurisdictions. The same regulations that apply to the traditional brick-and-mortar and mail-order pharmacies typically apply to online pharmacies."

The National Association of Boards of Pharmacy doesn't regulate on-line pharmacies, but it has developed a national "seal of approval" system that involves thoroughly investigating on-line pharmacies and giving them a Verified Internet Pharmacy Practice Sites (VIPPS) seal of approval. The VIPPS organization is made up of the pharmacy boards from fifty states, the District of Columbia, three U.S. territories, nine Canadian provinces, and four Australian states.

Every pharmacy that applies for VIPPS certification gets an on-site inspection.

It's no surprise that the legitimate on-line pharmacies lined up for inspection and approval so they could display the VIPPS logo. Sites that do not require a physician's prescription and do not have a pharmacist available for consultation need not apply.

These bogus online pharmacies try to get around the physician's role by stating that, in lieu of a preexisting relationship with a physician and a physical checkup, all the patient has to do is fill out a questionnaire. The state boards of pharmacy and the American Medical Association reject this "questionnaire" dodge as potentially dangerous and totally unprofessional. The FDA also opposes use of the questionnaire by online pharmacies. It's just not safe: Some prescription drugs are too dangerous for anyone to take who isn't being monitored by a physician.

Then there is the question of privacy. You may not want strangers to know what drugs you are taking and other personal details. These "medicine men" can sell your name to other, possibly illegitimate, vendors. These fraudulent pharmacies often sell names off their lists to individuals and companies marketing counterfeit products and deceptive services.

Many online pharmacies that rely on e-mail advertising to millions through purchased mailing lists feature just a few so-called "lifestyle" drugs. These drugs promise to treat such conditions as impotence, weight loss, chronic pain, and scarring acne. The VIPPS people suggest that this type of ad could be an instant giveaway that you're not dealing with reliable merchants. These drug sites may grab your attention and offer to solve all your problems, but they aren't regulated, they generally don't deliver what they say they will, and you're flirting with danger if you deal with them.

If you are searching for a reliable online pharmacy, try the VIPPS Web site at www.nabp.net for suppliers that will meet your needs.

## BUYING ONLINE FROM CANADA

The American dollar is strong in Canada. Chapter 14 explains how actually traveling across the border can be remarkably cost-efficient for prescription drug customers, but what about buying online from Canadian sources?

Canadian pharmacies are enjoying a boom in drug sales from American customers, but what's the best way to find out who's legitimate and who isn't? While

VIPPS includes representatives from Canada, it is not empowered to regulate Canadian online sites. It's likely that VIPPS will eventually collaborate with Canadian authorities so that its seal of approval may apply to the country's legitimate pharmacies. But until it does, another organization, made up of private citizens, has taken on the job of checking out individual Canadian pharmacies with on-site inspections.

It's called the Internet and Mail Order Pharmacy Accreditation Commission (IMPAC). Some legitimate Canadian pharmacies are backing IMPAC, which has its headquarters in Manchester, Vermont. IMPAC is made up of pharmacists and physicians from the United States and Canada who have banded together to work out a VIPPS-like pharmacy inspection routine, according to David D. Mackay, who works for CanadaDrug.com, one of the founding members. (The FDA reportedly does not officially approve of IMPAC because it is not a government-sanctioned organization.)

Mackay says IMPAC inspectors go into Canada and check out each applicant pharmacy on site. If the checklist is clean, then the pharmacy gets IMPAC's stamp of approval. While this does not provide a true government approval, as

## Left to Your Own Devices?

Millions of consumers are buying medical products on the Internet—putting themselves at risk by purchasing medical devices without prescription or proper fittings. According to the FDA Center for Devices and Radiological Health, contact lenses are sold on the Internet without a prescription, as well as hearing aids, which should be selected and fitted by health-care professionals. The FDA says that some sites have even offered artificial hearts.

Other devices being sold online may not hurt you anywhere but in the pocketbook, but unwitting shoppers may be bankrupting themselves by purchasing an endless array of items such as magnets, copper appliances, and more to "cure" arthritis.

If a device is labeled in many languages or carries measurements in metric units, it may not be licensed for sale in the United States or meet U.S. safety requirements. The market for "miracle cure-alls" has found a new home online, but you don't have to be a victim.

VIPPS does, it's a lot better than nothing. The practice of Americans buying American drugs from Canadian pharmacies is expanding, even as the major pharmaceutical companies oppose it at every turn. If you'd like to check out what popular prescription drugs cost in Canada as compared with the U.S., go to www.affordableRx.com.

## How to Buy Online Safely

You're now a well-informed consumer who understands the challenges of purchasing your prescription drugs online. You've been warned about the charlatans, you've been alerted to dangerous practices, and you know how to identify risky Web sites.

Now—how do you actually do it?

First comes the research. You diligently look up and check out online pharmacies, and you know you can get a good price for your prescription medicines. You're confident you are dealing with a dependable supplier. You're ready to order.

But no reliable online pharmacy will touch your order without a valid prescription from your physician. So how do you get this written, hard copy prescription into an electronic, online system?

It's easy. The first time you don't even try. You do things the old-fashioned way by having your physician phone or fax in the prescription. State laws usually require prescriptions to be faxed from your physician's office, not your home or office. Security is assured this way. A pharmacist must verify the existence of an actual, physician-signed prescription.

But this isn't as fast as walking across the street to CVS. Buying prescription drugs from an online pharmacy is best when you're dealing with a chronic or semi-chronic condition, for which you need ongoing medication. It isn't recommended for one-shot medicines that you need right away, such as antibiotics.

Once your online pharmacy has received your physician's prescription and filed it, you're ready to go. The Web site will ask you to fill out an order form, provide a shipping address, and supply credit card information. You will receive a confirming e-mail that provides a projected delivery date and an order number.

Ordering refills is easy. You can e-mail your prescription request at your convenience, always allowing enough shipping time for the refill to arrive. If you have questions, you can dial a toll-free number and confer with a pharmacist. You can e-mail questions and get them answered, often within a day or two. You can request that a "patient profile" of all the medicines you are taking be created, and you can update it as needed.

You can also use the company's toll-free number to order your refills, but on-line orders generally go through more quickly. There's no waiting for a busy pharmacist to answer your phone call. The first few times, it may feel a little strange to order your prescription in this way, but you may soon love its convenience—as Mary Ellen did.

A seventy-nine-year-old widow, Mary Ellen lives in an apartment and regularly takes four prescription drugs. Getting to a pharmacy requires a taxi ride or getting a lift from a friend. A volunteer at her senior center told her about ordering online and helped her get started. Now Mary Ellen uses the laptop computer her son gave her as a birthday present to order her prescription drugs and has them mailed to her home free of charge. (She also uses her laptop to order DVDs from Netflix, shop at QVC.com, and participate in a Weight Watchers online support group!)

## WHY BUYING IN-HOME TESTS ONLINE CAN BE RISKY

Pills aren't the only pharmaceutical product for sale on the Internet. You can also purchase home tests for pregnancy, fertility, HIV, hepatitis, cholesterol, blood sugar, and more. Some test kits promise to detect the presence of illegal drugs such as marijuana, amphetamines, nicotine, or methamphetamines in your children or your employees.

If the tests are available over the counter, then you can buy them online from a reliable pharmacy without concern for their safety. But some tests sold on-line are illegal and others are not FDA-approved. Many in vitro diagnostic tests have been cleared for professional use only in your health-care provider's office. Some of the tests require follow-up tests to confirm the results. Others, such as the test to screen for prostate cancer that looks for PSA (prostrate surface antigen), must be paired with a rectal examination and more detailed testing if a positive result turns up.

The FDA Center for Devices and Radiological Health suggests a few red flags that should alert you to unreliable products and sellers. *Don't buy the test* if it:

- Claims to diagnose more than one illness, such as cancer, arthritis, and anemia

- Is made in a country other than the United States (even if made in the United States, buy it *only* if the FDA has cleared or approved the test for use at home)

- Is made by only one laboratory and sold directly to the public (this is not intended for over-the-counter sale)

Other red flags that should raise immediate concerns, according to the FDA, include claims that the government or medical profession are "conspiring" to block the product and tests and mark the drug for export only.

Staff at the FDA, working with the Federal Trade Commission, and the National Consumer League's Fraud Information Center, monitor Internet offers and promise to take action against those with misleading marketing or unsafe products. This includes warning letters demanding that site owners stop selling such medical devices unless they can prove the FDA has cleared or approved them for sale.

If you have questions or complaints about a particular medical device or Web site, you can call the FDA at (888) INFO-FDA or your local FDA district office. They can tell you if the FDA has cleared or approved the medical device you're checking on. You can also report false claims to the Federal Trade Commission (FTC) at (877) FTC-HELP.

## THE FUTURE FOR ELECTRONIC PRESCRIPTION

The end may be in sight for the familiar physician's prescription notepad, which may be replaced by software designed to send prescription orders to pharmacies electronically. One such service offered by SureScripts requires a physician to punch in code information, which is then sent electronically to a pharmacist at an online or local pharmacy. It's all part of a high-tech loop that will make sending prescriptions and getting your medicine much easier for all concerned. And there won't be any more mix-ups because of physicians' famously wretched handwriting.

If you're uncertain about what to do in your quest for the best medicine at the best price, check online pharmacies to compare prices and see how things work.

The chain drugstore list on page 147 is a good place to start. Also look at www.Drugstore.com and the National Community Pharmacy Association's www.CornerDrugstore.com (this group represents independent drugstores). The site at www.PillBot.com compares prices quoted by all of the major on-line pharmacies for any prescription drug in various doses and for different numbers of pills.

Buying prescription drugs on the Internet is a practice that is clearly here to stay. You need to practice caution, but consider giving this twenty-first-century system a try.

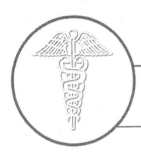

## FOURTEEN

## CROSSING THE BORDER

Buying online works for many people, but not everyone feels comfortable dealing with an unseen pharmacist, using the Internet to purchase by credit card, or waiting for prescription drugs to come in the mail. The good news is that other options exist, but at least one requires leaving home and travelling to another country.

Prescription drug buyers who make these journeys have launched a new kind of American revolution. Like the Sons of Liberty, who in 1773 protested unfair taxation by dumping over three hundred crates of tea, prescription drug users today are protesting high drug costs by driving into Canada and Mexico in search of affordable drugs. They just want a fair price, and it's well worth the time and cost of the trip.

This chapter explains how this phenomenon began, what the legal issues are, and how to join the "exodus" yourself, no matter where in the country you live. You'll discover just how easy it can be to save hundreds, even thousands, of dollars on the drugs you take every day.

### IN THE BEGINNING

It started back in the nineties with a few pioneers who discovered that they could get American-made prescription drugs in Canada for almost half the price of the same medication at home. When word got out, what began as a trickle of people making occasional visits to our northern neighbor soon turned into a stream of shoppers choosing regular road trips instead of going bankrupt trying to keep up with ever-rising prescription costs.

Who were these hardy individuals? Some were frustrated seniors struggling to pay for their multiple prescriptions; others had used up their savings to treat a sick child. All were willing to be part of the first experiments in purchasing drugs outside the United States.

In 1995 the first organized prescription drug trip left St. Paul, Minnesota, which is about three hundred miles from the Canadian border. Kate Stahl, eighty-four, a retired medical secretary, remembers the excitement and camaraderie among the members of that first trip across the border to Winnipeg, Manitoba, in Canada.

"I went along with my husband, who needed a half dozen different meds. We went up on a bus, and the trip took three days and two nights. We felt like pioneers, like we were showing the way.

"One of the staffers with the Minnesota Senior Federation, the trip's sponsor, had lived in Winnipeg and knew people who worked for the Medimart Pharmacy there," Stahl says. "Initial inquiries turned into serious negotiations for drug purchases.

"We chartered a big Greyhound bus because school buses just wouldn't do for such a long trip." She recalls the sense of excitement among the passengers. "We sang some songs, chatted a lot, and just felt we were having a lot of fun.

"The whole trip only cost sixty dollars a person (not including the drugs)," Stahl says, smiling at the memory. The senior federation was able to negotiate some free hotel and meal stops with various casinos along the way to help defray the costs. "I think the casinos were interested in us because they cater to seniors who have the time and the money to gamble," Stahl says.

Several years later the busloads got bigger and expenses mounted. The federation was running out of funds to operate the trips. That's when U.S. Senator Mark Dayton, a Minnesota Democrat whose family founded the Dayton store chain, stepped in to subsidize the trips with his own money. His motives were described as both humane and political. He wanted to help the Minnesota seniors continue saving money on their prescription drugs, but he also wanted to use the bus trips as a political tactic to demonstrate a growing problem: that

Americans were paying a lot more at home for the same American-made drugs sold in Canada.

Some of those who joined the bus trips initially now prefer to make the trip in their own cars. But for new members and those who prefer to leave the driving to others, the bus trips continue. They're strategically organized so riders first go to Canada and establish a relationship with the pharmacy there. Then they can have refills sent to them by mail. It's a highly organized plan that corporate purchasing agents would probably admire. But problems do exist. Refills run out and new prescriptions have to be hand delivered to the pharmacies, and the weather can be a problem.

"We really can't go into Canada during the winter months because it's just too cold and the roads are hazardous," Stahl says. So the Minnesota Senior Federation worked out a solution. On the last trip in late October, members get a three-month prescription drug supply with three refills. That will get them through the winter. When they run out of refills they have to get a new prescription from their doctor and make another trip to Canada.

Peter Wyckoff, the federation's executive director, says that its members still take five to seven trips a year during the warmer months, enjoying the singing and socializing that make the travel time pass quickly. He notes that even with the mail-order program, many federation members still choose to take the bus trips to Canada because they prefer to see a pharmacist face to face. This way, he adds, they get a trained professional to answer their questions and to make sure they are not buying drugs that will conflict with other medications they take.

While most participants considered the first trips into Canada an adventure, for many the necessary subsequent sorties became a burden. Many Minnesota border-crossers resent going into Canada to get their prescriptions for a reasonable price instead of at home. "It's unconscionable," Stahl says, "and it's a disgrace that citizens in a country as big as ours have to put up with this."

Until the prices go down or the laws change, the federation plans to continue its efforts. Recently it did a price comparison, checking the cost of Canadian drugs against those in the United States. They shopped a market basket of thirteen commonly prescribed drugs, including Celebrex (for arthritis relief), Tamoxifen (cancer), Lipitor (cholesterol), Nexium (acid reflux disease), and Synthroid (hormone deficiency). A ninety-day supply of the thirteen medicines came to an average of $2,052 when priced at American chain drugstores. The federation was able to deliver from Canada the same size supply of the same drugs for only $774, a whopping 62 percent savings.

The Minnesota federation is making its low-cost, reimported drugs from Canada available to "anyone in this country who needs help," Stahl says. To find out more information, see the Appendix.

## New England Prescription

New England, home of the Boston Tea Party, Paul Revere's ride, and all those Minutemen, turns out to be a hotbed of prescription revolutionaries. While Minnesota seniors may have taken the first bus trip across the border, New Englanders were not far behind. (It's not so surprising when you consider that the state motto of New Hampshire is Live Free or Die.) Russell W. E. Woodard, seventy-three, a Pierpont, New Hampshire, retired field supervisor with a milk cooperative, made his first trip into Canada four years ago. It was covered by a CBS *60 Minutes* TV crew as a political and personal finance story.

Woodard and his wife, Suzanne, now seventy, took an organized bus ride to Montreal, where they found typical Canadian savings of 40 to 50 percent. "This was a real break for us," Woodard says, "because we were paying more than $700 a month for the two of us to cover medicine for cholesterol, prostate cancer, bladder cancer, diabetes, and heart disease."

The Woodards learned that prices in Canada are well below what they are in the United States because the Canadian government controls prescription drug prices. They also benefited from a favorable exchange rate for the U.S. dollar. Initially the Woodards were able to purchase a six-months' supply of their prescribed drugs. But, he says, "the American pharmaceutical companies raised such a fuss, the limit was reduced to a three-months' supply."

For their first trip, Woodard says, each prescription was written by his doctor and then faxed to a pharmacist in Montreal. The pharmacist had a Canadian physician rewrite it on his prescription pad so the pharmacy could accept it. But the second time around, Woodard says, "a Canadian doctor had to meet with us, to check out why we were taking the drugs, before he wrote the prescription." Now, he adds, the routine is much smoother.

"We have five children and six grandchildren, and it got to a point where we were having to go without most of our medicines because the prices were going over our heads," Woodard says. "These trips to Canada saved our lives, physically and financially." He and Suzanne have become embittered about what they maintain is "way too much power in the hands of the drug companies." He scoffs at rumors and reports from the drug companies that seek to deter Americans from buying drugs in Canada. The reports he refers to suggest that Canadian medicine might be contaminated. "They get exactly the same drugs we have here," he says. The Woodards are still taking the bus trips north.

## THE LEGAL ISSUES

"Buying prescription drugs from other countries and bringing them into the United States is called *drug importation*," says the American Pharmaceutical Association. "Drug importation is illegal. Many health-care professionals (including pharmacists) are concerned about drug importation because it can be very dangerous to your health." Customs officials, however, have historically overlooked the practice when it involves Americans bringing back a three-months' supply of prescription drugs for their personal use. You show your prescription and your drug purchases and they waive you by with an understanding nod.

To date, no American has been forced to relinquish the prescription drugs they bought for personal use (accompanied with a proper prescription) when crossing into the United States. According to Lee Graczyk, spokesman for the St. Paul-based Senior Federation, "U.S. Customs personnel are just not enforcing the letter of the law."

Because border-crossers can save an average of 40 percent on their drug purchases in Canada and Mexico, the American pharmaceutical companies are trying to put the squeeze on Canadian pharmacy wholesalers by saying export deliveries could be cut back by the amount of drugs that are going to Americans. It's a hardball game. But, as it's being played out, Americans, by the thousands, continue to take advantage of the big price breaks you can get across the border.

## CONSIDER HEADING TO MEXICO

For many Americans, Mexico is simply a tourist destination, a land of bullfights and mariachi bands, where a tropical climate, charming villages, and beautiful beaches attract visitors all year long.

But for Americans who live on or near the border, Mexico has also become known as a paradise for prescription drug bargains. Initially, this was a well-kept secret among ranchers and other residents who live along "the line" with Mexico. Now the word has gotten out—alerting thrifty seniors and other prescription drug buyers who don't live anywhere near the country's southern border. Go to Mexico, they hear through this information pipeline. You can have a good time shopping and pick up a three-months' supply of prescription drugs for a fraction of what you have to pay back home.

Alan C. Gotland and his wife Jan are comanagers of Circle Z Ranch in Patagonia, Arizona. Nogales, a major border town, is just fifteen miles away. Being able to buy prescription drugs on the Mexican side of the border, Gotland says, is almost like having insurance coverage, because drug prices are so low.

"My doctor prescribed an expensive maintenance drug for a skin condition on my toes, but I nearly fainted when I learned that it would cost me $648," he says. Then Gotland's doctor told him not to worry because he could have his prescription filled for a lot less money in one of the Mexican border pharmacies.

Gotland went into Nogales, Mexico, and headed to a four-block area where all the *farmacias* are located. They're not at all like American pharmacies, he notes. They are relatively small stores that sell only prescription drugs, which are lined up along rows and rows of shelves. There's no shampoo or soap, no magazines, candy, or other consumer products that usually dominate American drugstores. These *farmacias* sell prescription drugs, nothing else.

When he placed his first order, Gotland was stunned at the price: just $110 for a three-months' supply.

How does it work? Gotland says that the sequence of events is always the same. When he's ready to cross the border back into the United States at the U.S. Customs inspection gate, he has to declare that he is bringing a drug product into the country. He also has to produce his American doctor's prescription to demonstrate that his purchase is for his own use.

That's all there is to it—no fuss, no muss, just a huge discount off what he would have to pay in an American pharmacy. But Gotland wonders why this huge savings is possible, why pharmaceutical companies in business to make a profit sell their products in Mexico for retail prices that are so much lower than those they charge a few miles across the border in the United States. "Something's wrong here," he says.

## BUT IS IT SAFE?

The pharmaceutical companies, trying to stem the tide of Americans crossing the border to buy drugs in Mexico, have publicized the likelihood that drugs purchased in a *farmacia* might be counterfeit or might contain unknown and potentially dangerous ingredients. While these companies raise some of the same concerns about Americans buying drugs in Canada, the public seems to take those warnings less seriously. Why? Because the Canadian government has such a good record of oversight when it comes to regulating the sale of prescription drugs to its own citizens.

But Mexican government regulations and inspections don't compare with Canada's. The most reliable "inspectors" for medicines sold in Mexico may be the thousands of Americans who regularly shop there. Although the *farmacias* are just bare counters, "all the drugs you buy are in the manufacturers' original sealed boxes and bottles with the proper dosage, warnings and expiration date on the label," says Gotland.

These days, it's not just border people like the Gotlands who are buying drugs in Mexico. Back when they lived in Phoenix, a four- to five-hour drive from Nogales, their doctor first advised them about the Mexican prescription connection. They decided they would make a day of it, so after they picked up their prescriptions they spent a few hours shopping and having a late lunch before heading home again. Because the Gotlands saved so much money, they decided the long drive wasn't a problem but an opportunity. They continued to make regular trips across the border, and they found plenty of ways to have fun while they were at it.

Now they host a variety of ranch guests, including many who combine a vacation with a trip to Mexico for regular prescription refills. Occasionally guests will also need to pick up an expensive antibiotic, such as Amoxicillin, and expresses amazement at how much they can save on whatever they need. Those who are new to border crossing for prescription drugs are given directions about where to go in Nogales. The Gotlands added that hordes of recreational vehicle owners also appear to know about buying low-cost drugs in Mexico, as traffic in town has measurably increased. They also noted that they haven't heard any stories of problems with the system or with buyers getting compromised drug products.

## DOUBLE YOUR BORDER BARGAINS

Some Americans have decided to double up on prescription drug savings while enjoying the splendors of the changing seasons. Betty Beverly, sixty-one, who lives in Helena, Montana, is the executive director of the Montana Senior Citizens Association. She says some of her association members have the best of both worlds. They get their prescriptions filled in the nearby Canadian province of Alberta during the warm weather. Then when the temperature grows cold, they join the "snowbirds" who go south for the winter. They avoid harsh winters and deep snow by traveling to Arizona, where they spend the colder months under clear skies and lots of sunshine.

Each summer, Beverly reports, Montana members from all over the state journey together up to Canada, as long as five hours each way. Like their cohorts in Arizona and other southwestern states, they view the trips as minivacation days full of fun, shopping, and lunching after they visit pharmacies for their prescriptions.

The prescription pilgrimages started out as chartered bus rides. Later, members began using their own cars because it was just more convenient. Instead of having to keep to a schedule or adjust to the group's needs, they were free to do their own thing. "Once we learned where to go and how it worked," Beverly says, "we struck out on our own."

Association members who pioneered the border-crossing trips say they refused to succumb to the "fear campaigns" organized by the drug companies. Instead, they viewed the warnings about the potential dangers of buying drugs in foreign countries as marketing propaganda. Even when they heard that it was possible to pick up a counterfeit drug or one that had been adulterated, they shook their heads and kept heading north.

"Our seniors are smart consumers—they're not stupid," says Beverly. She says there have not been "any newspaper, magazine, or TV stories about American seniors becoming ill or dying from drugs they purchased in Canada."

## THE QUESTION PEOPLE KEEP ASKING

It's difficult to understand why the United States allows this situation to continue. Why must citizens have to cope with wildly inflated prescription drug prices by traveling to Canada or Mexico to find prices they can afford? "It's a disgrace that we've come to this," says Woodard, the New Hampshire border-crosser. His feelings are echoed by thousands of Americans who suffer "sticker shock" every time they pick up a prescription at their local pharmacies.

The number of border-crossers is growing. In some places the practice has evolved to include easier arrangements with Canadian pharmacies to provide mail-order delivery for drug purchases made online. For many seniors and those who are frail or otherwise unable to travel great distances, these Canadian "connections" provide a tremendous financial boon.

It is becoming more and more clear to Americans that they are the only people on this continent overpaying for their medications. How is it that the pharmaceutical companies can sell their drugs at a much lower rate in Canada and Mexico than in the U.S? Why should U.S. citizens be the ones to foot the bill to subsidize drugs being sold over the border? The level of anger and frustration has grown. Instead of passively accepting the drain on their finances, people are complaining to their representatives.

## CAUTION: BUY FROM TRUSTED SOURCES

Prescription drug counterfeiters operate in this country and elsewhere. These crooks are slick. They can make fake pills look like the originals and design their packages to look just the same. Caches of counterfeit drugs have been found in Mexico and Canada—and in the United States. This is why savvy customers only patronize pharmacies that have proven over the years to be reliable.

How can you find trustworthy sources for your discounted medicines? Your best bet is talking to the people who've been buying regularly for years. Check with members of local senior clubs, ranchers, merchants in border towns, respected physicians, and others familiar with the area you're visiting. Buying drugs across the border can and should be a win-win proposition. Steady customers keep a business healthy and provide a stream of new customers to these border pharmacies. It's in their best interest to serve you well and provide a reasonably priced and safe product.

## CANADIAN MAIL-ORDER BUYING MOVES TO BROOKLYN

The *New York Daily News* reported on October 15, 2003, that a Canada-based Internet seller had opened a mail-order store in Brooklyn—the first outlet in the city to offer "inexpensive drugs from north of the border." Best Canadian Pharmacy Service is an "independently owned American agent" for LePharmacy Inc. of Montreal.

The company hopes to attract thrifty drug buyers who may not have Internet access or who may not be comfortable ordering drugs online. The owner of the shop, Jacqueline Feldman, notes that consumers "will save up to 80 percent." She adds, "Pharmaceutical companies are making a killing every year. I'm hoping what I'm doing will allow people who are older or sick and need to be on a maintenance medication to save some money."

The company hopes to open as many as fifteen stores in the greater New York City area, and Mark Lazar, CEO of LePharmacy.com, promises that the drugs sold will be the best. "The only difference in the drugs in Canada and the U.S. is the label," he said.

The *News* article went on to quote an FDA spokesman who said he knew of no complaints lodged against the company and that state authorities are not likely to get involved. "As long as [the state attorney general's] office is convinced that New York State consumers are not being defrauded or medically harmed, it's not very likely that we're going to take strong action to close these places down," said Marc Violette, a spokesman for state Attorney General Eliot Spitzer.

Stay tuned—companies like this one may be coming your way.

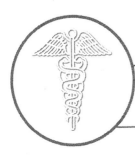

**FIFTEEN**

## Discount Deals

Are you independently wealthy, a recent lottery winner, or a major stockholder in one of the big pharmaceutical companies? Probably not, because you bought this book to learn how to save money on prescription drugs. You don't want to pay a cent more for your medications than you have to.

The magic word is *discount*—which is simply a price below the listed or announced price.

Who gets these discounts? Could you qualify for some terrific price cut that you've never heard of before? This chapter introduces you to some of the ways you can save money on your prescription medications right here in the U.S.A., at drugstores right in your neighborhood. All you need is one of the many discount cards offered to consumers who meet particular requirements.

There are literally hundreds of these discount cards and special purchase deals, and they promise to help cut your prescription drug costs from 15 to 40 percent. Even better, if you or a family member has a very limited income, there are programs that will provide prescription drugs at no charge.

You may be surprised to learn that many major drug companies offer discount deals on certain medications. So do membership organizations such as AARP. Various states offer special purchase programs for their residents, but you also may qualify if you visit a doctor in that state and receive a prescription during your visit. The Department of Veterans Affairs offers discounts to qualified veterans of all the armed forces. Some days it seems that everywhere you look, someone is offering you a discount deal.

But you need to be clear about what each discount actually represents in savings. While every discount offer may save you something off the retail price of a prescription drug, does anyone really pay the "retail" price? For example, suppose a drug company offers you a discount card that promised to save you 15 percent off every prescription. If you would normally pay a retail price of $280 for a thirty-day supply of your medicine, when you present the discount card, you pay $238—a savings of $42. That's fine, as far as it goes.

But you could buy the same drug from a Canadian pharmacy at 40 to 50 percent off, and save far more. Or you might be able to get a generic equivalent for considerably less. In some instances an over-the-counter product can provide the same therapeutic effect for a fraction of the cost.

With so many different options available and so many different discounts offered, it can be difficult to make sense of all the facts and figures. Finding the discount program that is right for your needs is the key to getting the most for your money.

## How Can You Find a Good Discount Plan?

When it comes to buying prescription drugs, your best sources for expert advice are your health-care partners: your pharmacist and physician. In many cases these pros can help you develop a cost-containment plan. They may also recommend sources you haven't considered for useful discount cards. If you're a senior, your local government should include agencies whose mandate is providing care for "elders" or "the aging." Don't be insulted by the terminology. Think of yourself as a member of a large and vocal voting bloc that makes up in experience and knowledge what it may lack in cash. Your taxes fund these offices, so it's more than reasonable to expect that they'll deliver on a promise of help. A good place to see if you can find discount plans is www.benefitscheckup.org, which is operated by the National Council on Aging. You fill in a questionnaire that includes such things as the drugs you are taking, your income level, and where you live. It's the easiest way to get started. The prescription benefits search includes all the drug company discount programs and a whole list of others. If you don't have a computer connection to the Internet, head for your local library or senior center. You won't be the only person doing this kind of on-line research, so you'll be able to ask for help. Or get your family involved—a grandchild who's a computer whiz may be just the right partner in digging up the best deals on discount cards.

## WHAT DOES IT TAKE TO QUALIFY?

Discount cards have all sorts of qualification rules. Generally, the steeper the card's discount, the more qualifications you must meet. Qualifiers for membership may include age, income, specific types of illnesses, or where you live.

You usually won't qualify *if you have insurance coverage that includes prescription drugs,* even if it's quite limited. Income limits vary from program to program, but most allow petitioners to have incomes at 200 percent of the poverty level, around $18,000 a year for singles and $24,000 a year for couples. These limits vary from plan to plan, as some allow higher incomes for special illness cases.

Some cards require annual fees for membership. For example, the AARP prescription card costs $19.95 a year per person. So a couple would pay $39.80 a year—there's no break for being married. The ProCare Card used by some chain drugstores costs $5 to enroll and $15.95 a month. Unless you have a medical condition that requires taking several costly drugs on a regular basis, you may not save much, if any, money with these.

## LOW-INCOME PATIENT
## ASSISTANCE PROGRAM

If you're barely surviving financially, your best hope will be to qualify for one of the major drug companies' Patient Assistance Programs (PAPs), which make prescription drugs available free to very low-income individuals. If you pass their income test, which mirrors the one used by most state discount card plans ($18,000 per year for singles and $24,000 for couples) and you're not eligible for any other assistance plan, you still may face an array of other hurdles. Your physician or one of the medical staff must complete a set of forms that are then forwarded to the drug manufacturers. These applications usually require copies of your most recent income tax returns.

Don't expect a speedy answer to your application for one of these programs.

Patients often have to wait many weeks for approval. Some companies will allow you a three- to four-month supply while you're waiting for confirmation, but you shouldn't expect assistance for any medication you need to take right away. Apply as soon as possible to take advantage of the program.

Do you need help in paying for three, four, even five drugs? If so, you may have to fill out an application for each one. There's also a time limit. Some companies make you reapply every three months and some every year, but if you're eligible, it can make the difference between survival and ongoing struggle.

Most physicians' offices, local government agencies, senior centers, and the like know the drill and can help you or even do most of the work for you. Don't let false pride get in the way—if you can get help to cut all the red tape, this PAP can be of great value. It can cut your prescription costs from hundreds of dollars a month to zero. And if you're below the income level, you may be eligible for a PAP, offered by the different drug companies, where you show your card and get your prescription purchase free.

These PAP deals can be lifesavers for low-income patients who must take several different drugs. Be aware that you can still qualify for some PAPs if your annual income is as high as $28,000 (or even higher) if you have one or more long-term illnesses. For more information about the PAP and other programs go to www.rxassist.org.

## PHARMACEUTICAL COMPANY DEALS

All of the major pharmaceutical companies offer a discount card, which allows you to purchase specific products at a reduced price. How do you find out about these cards? Check your physician's office for brochures that explain what discounts are available for that company's drugs.

You're likely to find two kinds of deals offered. One type gives you 15 percent or more off the listed price when you show the card to your pharmacist. The other sort allows you to pay a flat fee—perhaps $12–$15—for any listed product, no matter what retail price is quoted.

Here's an example: Pfizer's Living Share Card lets you buy a thirty-day supply of its medications for only $15 each, but you must qualify for this card by meeting specific income criteria. Also you have to keep reapplying for the capped price

## Sample Pharmaceutical Discount Card Programs

A number of pharmaceutical companies have banded together to offer a discount program, called the "Together Card", which works for all of their prescription drug products as a convenient way to handle the situation of high prices. The initial companies that formed the Together Rx Card program are Abbott Laboratories, AstraZenica, Aventis, Bristol-Myers Squibb, GlaxoSmithKline, Jansen Pharmaceuticals, Novartis and Ortho-McNeil. When you see the Together Card logo, you can expect discounts of anywhere from 15 to 40 percent off retail prices for more than 170 medicines. Go to the card's Web site (www.TogetherRx.com) or call 1-800-865-7211 for more information.

### ELY LILLY AND COMPANY

The "Lilly Answers Card" limits your cost for a monthly supply to $12. Call (877) RX-LILLY or go to www.lillyanswers.com.

### GLAXOSMITHKLINE

Using the "Orange Card" discounts saves you from 15 to 40 percent, depending on the prescription product. Call (888) ORANGE6.

### NOVARTIS PHARMACEUTICAL COMPANY

The "Care Card" has discounts of 15 percent and up. Call (800) 865-7211 or go to www.careplan.novartis.com to find out how to use this card along with the Together Rx card.

### PFIZER

The "Living Share Card" lowers your payment to $15 for a thirty-day supply of the company's prescription products at participating pharmacies. Call (800) 717-6005.

every thirty days. So while this kind of low-cost, one-price deal is far better than just getting a 15 percent discount, it takes continued work on your part to get it.

## CHAIN STORE DISCOUNTS

Does your discount chain or "big box" superstore want you to buy your prescriptions there? Of course. Few people go to Costco and come home with a single item in a small paper bag. If Costco gets your prescription drug business, it's also likely you'll buy your groceries there. And while you're picking up your groceries, you might pick up a new computer printer and maybe price some tires for your car.

National and regional chain stores often provide discount programs for seniors, particularly those on a limited income. These aren't always advertised, so you may have to ask if a discount is available and what kinds of products are included. (Does it just cover prescription drugs, or can you save money on vitamins, herbal remedies, even healthy food products?) Are you a member of AARP? You're eligible as soon as you or your spouse turns fifty, and you certainly don't have to be retired. AARP offers its members a variety of money-saving discounts and alerts its members to many others through its newsletter and magazine.

Most of these programs specifically benefit seniors, but some are designed to help anyone on a lower income. Just remember: Is the discount you're getting the best price available for the product you need?

## STATE PROGRAM BARGAINS

Sometimes the best deals are homegrown—if you live in a state where the government has responded to consumer complaints about the high price of prescription drugs by offering state discount programs. These prescription discount programs benefit seniors and low-income families, and more states are joining the movement. There are primarily two kinds of plans:

### INCOME-BASED

At this writing, twenty-six states have established income caps for citizens who want to purchase drugs at subsidized prices. As a rule these programs are limited to individuals whose annual income is not more than $18,000 and not more than $24,000 for couples. Under certain circumstances, these limits can be raised because of a patient's medical condition. Income limitations may vary from state to state, but not by much.

### DISCOUNT CARDS

California, Florida, Iowa, New Hampshire, New York, Massachusetts, Ohio, and West Virginia currently offer a prescription drug discount card. Other states are hopping on the bandwagon every day. If your state isn't on this list, keep checking—and consider writing to your state legislators to ask for their help in launching a discount drug program. Check with your pharmacist, physician, and regional agency on aging to see when and if your state may offer such a card. Discounts vary, so you'll need to check with your state representatives. Some state discount programs require that you are sixty-five or older with a modest income—but not all. Here are a few specifics.

## DIVIDE AND CONQUER

The name of the game is *pill splitting*. For some medications, you can get a prescription for double your normal dose for the same price or a tiny bit more and then simply cut your pills in half, so if you've been taking a 25-milligram tablet, now you get 50-milligram doses, and cut them in half. Because most drugs cost very nearly the same no matter the dosage, you will usually save half the cost of your prescription by splitting the higher-dose pill.

The *Washington Post* reported, for instance, that thirty tablets of Zocor at CVS.com cost $129.99 for 20-milligram tablets—but only $129 for 40-milligram tablets! Viagra (at Eckerd.com) and Zoloft (at CVS.com) cost exactly the same for both dosage sizes, and Paxil (at Drugstore.com) and Celexa (Walgreens.com) ran only five dollars more for the double-sized dose.

Most physicians will agree to write a prescription for the double dosage, unless a patient might not be capable of doing the task correctly (because of some physical or mental limitation such as Parkinson's disease, tremors, advanced arthritis, or general frailty or confusion).

Drug manufacturers, however, warn that splitting pills could be dangerous, as do some major health insurers. Their reasons are logical: Patients might not do it the right way, and may end up taking less than a prescribed dose because a chunk or two crumbled and fell to the floor. Or patients might become confused and take the whole pill instead of half, "overdosing" on the higher dosage.

Note: Do *not* try to split capsules or coated tablets. The coating may protect the active ingredients from the harmful effects of stomach acid, or allow the active ingredients to release within the intestine so that it will not harm the stomach. And because pill splitting does not always give you two equal halves, it could be dangerous to split very potent medications. Ask if a capsule or a small pill comes in a larger tablet that can be split.

### CALIFORNIA AND FLORIDA

Discounts for anyone with a Medicare ID card, with savings from 15 to 40 percent.

### MASSACHUSETTS.

You are eligible as long as you fall under the income cap.

### NEW HAMPSHIRE

You have to be at least sixty-five, but there is no enrollment fee and no income limit.

### NEW YORK

Those sixty-five and older can get an Epic Card. Depending on income, you either pay for prescription drugs up to a certain deductible amount and then there's a cap on what you have to pay for your prescriptions or you pay a minimal annual fee and receive discounted drug prices.

### IOWA

A $20 enrollment fee is required.

Wherever you live, be aware that the rules in your state may change without much warning; also be warned that your discount benefits may change at any time. But let's be optimistic—perhaps they'll change in your favor. Your pharmacist and your physician's staff should be able to help you keep up with changes in the program.

## WHY EVERY DISCOUNT OFFER IS NOT A GOOD ONE

You've now learned about the many discount programs available to you from relatively familiar agencies, companies, and organizations. But you're likely to be invited to join many others, and you need to be aware that not every discount offer is a good one.

Imagine this: You're eating dinner one evening, and the phone rings. A pleasant, fast-talking person asks if you're having difficulty paying for your prescription drugs and offers first a sympathetic ear, then a fantastic medical discount card that will solve all your problems. You consider yourself a careful consumer, so you ask about the cost and a money-back guarantee. The caller says you'll save the cost of the card in just one month, and of course it's guaranteed.

If you're like thousands of other Americans, you may well say yes, sure, that sounds like the card for me. But if you do, you'll be the newest victim of a prescription drug scam that will cost you money and deliver almost no discounts worth having.

The *AARP Bulletin* recently profiled one of these scam artists, the Toronto-based MedPlan Inc., which charged people an annual fee of $340 but provided few useful drug discounts and, it turned out, no guarantee. The company is now under investigation by the FTC and by individual states on charges of unauthorized billing of credit and debit cards. The *Bulletin* reports that this one telemarketing company had gross receipts in 2002 of more than $8 million before the U.S. and Canadian governments shut it down and froze its assets.

The FTC Web site says these "fraudulent telemarketers" offer a plan to save money on prescription drugs, dental, vision, hearing, chiropractic, and nursing services. They may lead you to believe that they're affiliated with your insurance company, bank, or state government. But they're not. Some of these phony discount card issuers actually try to persuade you that the program they're offering is a substitute for health insurance. Patients who have been fooled into believing this are shocked to discover that no hospital or doctor's office will accept this fake "coverage."

Your warning is when they ask you to "confirm" your credit card or checking account number, implying that they already have this information—never fall for this. Simply hang up the phone.

Unfortunately, once these scam artists have your account information, they can charge your card for any amount they like. By the time you realize the problem, these companies have often changed their phone numbers or simply vanished.

As with all solicitations, your best protection is never to give out personal information on the phone or the Internet, especially (but not exclusively) financial information like credit card or bank account numbers—unless you originated the call to a company you know. By protecting your personal data, you are much less likely to become a victim of identity theft and other types of fraud.

If you fear that a telephone solicitor has "tricked" you into giving your credit card or bank account numbers, immediately call your bank or credit card issuer to block any unauthorized charges. Don't let embarrassment make the situation worse. Your report will be added to others in the FTC databases so that law enforcement officials can pursue these criminals both here at home and abroad. To file a complaint or to get free information on consumer issues, visit www.ftc.gov or call (877) FTC-HELP; TTY (866) 653-4261.

## THE ART OF THE DISCOUNT DEAL

When it comes to buying prescription drugs, your best sources for expert advice are your health-care partners, your pharmacist, and your physician. Also, area agencies on aging (in the phone book under county and city government headings) can help cut through the math so you can decide which discount offers the best deal for your particular situation.

This means learning all you can about discount programs available to you. Discounting is just one tactic, and you'll want to compare the benefits to other cost-cutting strategies, such as those described in chapters 13 and 14 about buying on-line or shopping across the border, or buying a less costly generic or over-the-counter equivalent.

Because many discount cards apply only to drugs made by specific companies, you need to know who makes the medicine your physician is prescribing. If you are taking several different drugs, you may have to apply for several manufacturers' cards. Be prepared to have and to use a whole deck of cards—it's just the way the game is played right now.

Shopping around, asking friends and family what works for them, and being open to a different strategy for each of your medications all contribute to money-saving success.

The important thing is to keep looking and keep asking for the help you need. If your income is close to qualifying you for free or deeply discounted medications, talk to someone who might be able to show you how to minimize your net income through accounting maneuvers. For this kind of help you may need to consult a professional who can help you with financial planning advice.

Stay in touch and on top of the situation. Join a local senior center or consider becoming a member of a local hospital association for seniors and former patients. Make it your business to follow politics and the news to be alerted to what may have changed in your favor. Just as a corporate purchasing agent may earn a bonus for finding the best prices on company supplies, you, too, will feel you've received a bonus when you locate the medicine you need at the best possible price. Success depends on remembering your *Smart Medicine* mantra: *Physician, Pharmacist, Patient.*

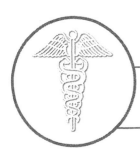

## SIXTEEN

# RUNNING TO COVERAGE

For many Americans, having health-care benefits that include prescription-drug coverage is crucial—and rightfully so. While illnesses requiring daily medication can occur at any time, more of these chronic conditions occur as we age. And these expenses can add up fast. It's not uncommon to have to take a half dozen pills a day. At more than four dollars a pill this could come to a $720 outlay every month—and even more if you have a partner who also has to take a multitude of drugs. Prescription horror stories are everywhere.

An increasing number of job seekers, especially older workers looking for second or third careers, put top priority on medical benefits with prescription coverage. "People who work for us tell us that their income is far less significant than their prescription-drug insurance coverage," says Larry E. Anderson, CEO of the National Older Worker Career Center in Arlington, Virginia.

It's not easy, Anderson says, because sometimes you have to search long and hard to find employers who have openings for jobs that provide health-care benefits. This is especially true when the economy is down and employers are cutting costs.

To fill employment gaps and keep costs down, employers may hire second- and third-career job seekers as part-time workers who are limited to fewer than twenty-five hours a week. When you work only part time, employers do not have to include you in their medical benefits plans.

For example, you can work three eight-hour days a week and not be qualified for benefits. The fast-food industry and many others often hire two people to fill one full-time job to avoid paying benefits.

## Consider This Career

Nurses are often in short supply—which means an increased demand for certified nursing assistants (CNAs) who work in hospitals, nursing facilities, clinics, other health-care venues, and in home care.

This career is proving popular among older folks. Not only does it generally offer prescription drug benefits, but you can take courses in area community colleges and become certified in a few months.

"We are seeing more older students in their fifties and sixties taking our CNA courses now," says Marilyn Leigh, RN, special projects coordinator with the Tarrant County College in Fort Worth, Texas.

For more information on CNA training and job opportunities, get in touch with your local community college and the various health-care facilities in your area (usually listed in the telephone book).

## PRESCRIPTION ENTREPRENEURS

If you're the boss of a small business or want to start up an enterprise of your own, home-based or otherwise, you have to face health insurance and prescription drug coverage head on. The sooner, the better. You may be spending money on equipment and services and putting off the health-care issue until later because it's too expensive right now. But the longer you put this off, the more dangerous your situation becomes.

You can join associations that cater to people like you who have specific skills and backgrounds. And the major health insurers have group policies that might fit your needs. Sometimes it's just a matter of biting the bullet and budgeting—making prescription coverage a priority.

Paul Edwards and wife Sarah, based in Pine Mountain Club, California, have made working at home an art form. Their books have become survival bibles for thousands of people who want to use stairways instead of highways for their commute. *Working From Home* (Tarcher/Putnam) has become a national best seller. Their more recent book, *Why Aren't You Your Own Boss?* (Prima/Random House), lists a variety of associations and organizations you may be able to join to qualify for group health insurance coverage.

"Unfortunately, a third of all self-employed people don't have any health insurance, and the number may be even greater when the next statistics come in," says Edwards. He and his wife enrolled with the Kaiser Permanente health maintenance organization to get the coverage they need. The prescription drug benefit, he says, costs around $200 a month but is well worth it: "If we pay $200 a month for the coverage and our drug costs would otherwise be more than $400 a month, it's quite a savings, isn't it?"

When you are a small business owner, he says, your company can provide you with a health-care benefit that pays for medical insurance expenses and medical bills that are not reimbursed. And, he says, any nonreimbursed medical bills, including prescription medicines, may qualify as a tax deduction. You should check this out with an accountant who specializes in small business tax matters.

## FIND THE ORGANIZATION THAT FITS

All kinds of associations, professional groups, and other such organizations provide medical benefits for members. By doing some research, you may be able to find an organization with group coverage that could save you considerable money on your prescriptions.

The AFTRA union, for example, offers insurance programs and medical coverage. For $250 per quarter, a family pays only $24 for a three-month supply of any brand name drug and only $9 for a three-month supply of any generic drug. A major mail-order drug warehouse supplier fills the prescriptions, and you can talk to a pharmacist on a toll-free number. A card gives a major discount at participating drugstore pharmacy counters, including all major chains.

Other associations, clubs, or groups offer member medical benefits with prescription coverage. Some coverage is better than others, so don't opt for the first plan that sounds good. But remember that almost any program is a lot better than none at all.

If you have any professional, artistic, or other specialized talent that can be a moneymaker, check out the Small Business Service Bureau at www.sbsb.com, where you can find a wide variety of organizations to query. Examples include the National Association of Self-Employed Silversmiths, home business associations, and associations for artists, crafts people, and female executives. For more information call (800) 343-0939. Web site libraries also have resource books with names, addresses, phone numbers, and descriptions of hundreds of associations, clubs, and other such entities.

## CONSIDER THE BIG ONES

Some of the major organizations, such as AARP, Department of Veterans Affairs, and a whole galaxy of college and university alumni associations, should be checked first. AARP has Medicare supplemental insurance for members who are sixty-five and above, covering prescription drugs up to $3,000 a year. Currently, you pay up to $210 a month for coverage, with a $250 deductible but no co-pay. For more information, call (800) 523-5800 or go to www.aarphealthcare.com. For members under age sixty-five, coverage is available but costs more.

### Do the Numbers

Before signing on for any benefit plan that covers prescription drugs, be sure that the monthly premiums, co-pays, and other costs don't add up to more than what you're actually paying for a year's worth of drugs. For example, Robert's association's plan includes prescription drug coverage. But he found that the program's monthly fee was nearly $250 and that there was a $300 deductible. He went over all his past year's prescription bills and discovered that he spent a monthly average of less than $250 on prescription medicines.

It made no financial sense for Robert to sign on with this health plan. He spent only about $250 per month on prescriptions, while with the plan he would pay fees of nearly $250 per month before buying any medicine—and he wouldn't get any prescription discounts until he'd spent $300.

Robert kept looking for a plan that better suited his needs.

## ATTENTION! VETERANS

You'd be surprised at how many men and women who served in the armed forces years back don't realize that they may be eligible for valuable medical coverage, including prescription drugs. If you qualify you can get a thirty-day supply of prescription drugs with a minimal co-pay of just $7 per prescription. And, unlike most other plans, the Department of Veterans Affairs coverage includes over-the-counter drugs. The cap on the co-pay plan is $840 a year, except for veterans with service-related injuries or conditions.

Here's how to find out if you qualify. Go to your nearest VA medical facility (hospital, clinic, and the like). You can find the names and phone numbers in your telephone book under "Veterans." Or check it out through your local American Legion or Amvets offices (also in the phone book). You first must enroll in the VA health-care program. More often than not, you'll be put on a waiting list, and it may take a few weeks before your application number comes up. There may be an income limit (although not for service-connected disabilities), and it can vary around the country. For more information, call (877) 222-VETS or go to www.VA.gov/elig/.

## CONSIDER UNIVERSITY MEDICAL PLANS

Colleges and universities around the country are using their alumni associations' group purchasing power to offer alumni and often their friends and families medical insurance that includes prescription drugs.

According to Steven Roy Goodman, a higher-education consultant based in Washington, D.C., many alumni associations are wooing new members and retaining others by offering hard-to-beat medical plans for those who do not have adequate coverage, or any coverage at all.

In some cases you have to ante up $100 or so to join, but often there's no charge. The bigger colleges and universities tend to offer better benefits, but most offer health-care coverage with minimal co-pays. You need not have graduated to be eligible. If you attended a college or university that has a plan that includes prescription coverage, you're in. As a matter of fact, you can be just about anybody these days to "qualify" for membership. What they're looking for is the biggest possible group in order to negotiate the best prices for members. Membership also includes such things as discounts on travel, purchasing a car, whatever. Benefit coverage lists are getting longer and longer.

Take the case of the University of Alabama National Alumni Association in Tuscaloosa, Alabama. According to Pat Whetstone, director of alumni affairs, association members are covered for prescription drugs with a modest co-pay. "There are no annual dues or fees, and anyone can participate . . . you don't have to be a graduate," he says. For more information, try the association's Web site at http://alumni.ua.edu. Check the area marked "Alumni Insurance Program."

Programs associated with some alumni associations may offer from 80 to 100 percent coverage, but you need to compare the premiums and what benefits are offered. Barbara, who just turned fifty, contacted her alumni association at Brandeis University and reviewed the details of the alumni health insurance programs described on its Web site. She reported that short-term insurance called GradMed provides coverage from 30 to 180 days for about $300 a month with a $250 deductible. But she found that the program was not available in some states (including New York, where she lived) and offered no coverage for prescription drugs or preventative care. It also did not cover gynecological checkups in all states.

Brandeis also offers its graduates access to AlumniMed+, a comprehensive health coverage plan described as covering many services, depending on your home state and the plan you select.

There are as many different kinds of programs as there are universities and colleges, so check around. You might become a "booster" who supports a particular institution and become eligible to participate in its health benefits programs.

## CHECK OUT UNIVERSITY RETIREMENT COMMUNITIES

A growing number of colleges and universities are attracting alumni and "friends" of the college to retire near the campus. By choosing to remain part of the university community, association members may be eligible for medical care, including prescription drugs, at an institution's hospital or clinic.

A retirement community called Capstone Village near the University of Alabama campus is planned for alumni, family members, and "friends" of the university. Residents are likely to have access to many university services, which may include medical coverage and prescriptions. Other universities in such states as Texas and Nebraska are looking to follow suit.

Penn State features The Village at Penn State, a life-care retirement community adjacent to the campus. The Village offers many amenities, including on-site assisted living and nursing care, though most residents are more interested in university cultural programs; athletic events; and a branch of the Penn State Creamery, which produces its own ice cream, sherbet, and cheeses.

If you live in a university town, you may want to explore the possibilities of allying yourself with the school for access to its medical benefits. Some areas may offer half a dozen options, so check around and choose what is best for you.

Check out your alma mater (or other colleges in areas where you might like to live) by visiting the university's Web site or by contacting the alumni association office by phone. (The main campus information phone number can connect you.)

## PRESCRIPTION WEDDING BELLS

When you marry later in life, financial planners suggest trust funds for each partner's children and estate planning. One thing that might be overlooked, and shouldn't be, is who has the medical insurance—and if the insurance includes prescription drug benefits.

Take the case of Millie Szerman, in her fifties, of Redondo Beach, California. She heads a little publishing venture and had some basic Blue Cross coverage that cost a hefty $400 a month. She had back surgery and some other major medical conditions that depleted her funds. She tried to change insurance companies but, with her medical history, she would have had to pay even more.

Then along came Jim, also in his fifties who had worked for a major hospital for more than twenty years before retiring. The two hit it off and decided to get married. The good news is that Jim is covered by his former employer's health plan, which includes prescription drugs for himself and his wife. Now the insurance will cover a second operation on her back and the handful of expensive pills she has to take daily.

Of course you wouldn't get married just to acquire health or prescription medication coverage—but it's a wonderful side benefit.

## GET HELP FROM THE GOVERNMENT

To qualify for Medicaid, a federal poverty level benefit administered by the states, your annual income must generally be below $8,980 for singles and $12,120 for couples. (This may differ from state to state.) Qualifying for Medicaid opens the way for getting prescription medications and nonprescription remedies at no cost. And if an older person, say, has very high prescription drug costs, it may be possible to get Medicaid relief even if you don't fall under the income limit.

Although Medicare does not yet provide significant prescription drug benefits, it pays under special circumstances. Medications will be covered under Medicare while you are confined in hospitals and for periods afterward under special situations, such as recuperating after transplant operations, according to Marisa Scala with the Center for Medicare Education in Washington. In other situations Medicare will cover drugs while you are in and out of the hospital. The discharge advisor can help you with this.

Many hospital patients are sent to nursing homes for recuperation and rehabilitation. There, Medicare will cover drug payments up to one hundred days. To

### A Benefits Tragedy

A retired Oklahoma City, Oklahoma, church official in his eighties suffers from a series of maladies including lupus, Parkinson's disease, and glaucoma, and has had recent heart surgery. His wife, also in her eighties, has had both cervical cancer and intestinal injuries caused by cobalt radiation treatment for the cancer. He takes ten prescribed pills each day, and his wife takes five different medications. Their drugs cost $1,200 each month.

The couple has supplemental Medicare coverage with Blue Cross, which provides a prescription drug benefit. But the insurance covers the couple for six months—and then the benefit cap stops the payments for the next six months until the next year opens up another six-month payment period. The couple lives on a modest pension and Social Security income plus some savings. Their resources are nearly gone, while the uncovered drug charges continue to rise. Their case resembles those of so many fixed-income retirees. Only a change in the Medicare drug benefit will prevent this ongoing tragedy from overwhelming this couple and others like them.

qualify you must have been confined in a hospital for at least three days and have a doctor's order for continuing care in a nursing facility. If injections have to be administered in a doctor's office, for such special needs as chemotherapy for cancer or medication for multiple sclerosis, Medicare will pay for it.

For people whose medical bills and other expenses are more than they can manage, the "spending down" Medicaid safety valve can help. If, for example, you have $800 monthly and the Medicaid eligibility cap is $600 monthly income, it may be possible to "spend down" income through paying medical bills to the point where Medicaid benefits will be guaranteed. More than 40 percent of older Americans have incomes of less than $20,000 a year and could be candidates for "spending down" to qualify for Medicaid. It's tricky and advice from a knowledgeable professional is a must. Call your area agency on aging for counseling. These agencies can usually be found in telephone book yellow pages or by calling the information operator.

## COBRA Benefits

If you lose your job, the law allows you to continue your employer-sponsored medical benefits, including prescription drugs, usually for eighteen months. It's all spelled out in federal government regulations mandated under a law called COBRA (Consolidated Omnibus Budget Reconciliation Act), which was passed in 1986.

This means employees can qualify for COBRA coverage by voluntary or involuntary termination of employment or by reduction in the number of working hours. If there is misconduct involved in the reason for getting fired, you won't be covered. In certain circumstances, the time limit may run longer than eighteen months in the case, say, of an employee's divorce when dependents have to be cared for.

The problem is that you have to pay your entire insurance premium, plus an administrative fee, and the costs can be prohibitive. However, it can be useful for the short term until you land another job with benefits or can find a more affordable health insurance plan. Before leaving your job, find out the exact costs, how to sign up, and when premiums are due. You should also be able to get information from your state or local department of labor.

## WHY YOU SHOULD RUN, NOT WALK

In a time when prescription drugs are often prohibitively expensive, everyone is helped by having some form of insurance coverage. If you work for a corporation that offers comprehensive medical benefits, you may be unaware of just what your benefits cover, but it's important to find out before you need them. Many young and middle-aged employees take their medical insurance for granted.

But medical problems often arrive without warning, and it's useful to know ahead of time what's available. You could develop a chronic illness such as rheumatoid arthritis and have to take very expensive drugs to maintain your mobility. You may never need a prescription filled for years at a time, then suddenly discover your child needs asthma medicine and inhalers whose cost adds up quickly.

If you're one of the many Americans between jobs or self-employed and have been "living on the edge" without prescription drug coverage, don't wait for financial disaster from a sudden need for expensive prescription medication to strike! Run, don't walk, and find some kind of protection as quickly as possible.

# TAKING BACK
# THE POWER

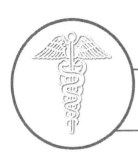

# SEVENTEEN

# ARE PRESCRIPTION DRUGS A LIFE SENTENCE?

We've spent most of this book talking about prescription drugs—what they are, who makes them, how to take them, how to buy them, and how to save money on them. So you may wonder about the title of this chapter. But if you *could* safely decrease your need for prescription medication, you would not only save money but benefit your health as well.

Many people wonder about the long-term effects of taking medication for a chronic condition. Some of the concerns involve the body's ability to use what it needs from a medication and "flush" the rest away without damaging vital internal organs. It's a sobering thought that a common over-the-counter medication such as Tylenol can cause liver ailments when consumed to excess. Even aspirin, which many have been encouraged to consume daily to help lower their risk of heart attacks, has caused stomach ulcers in people sensitive to the "acid" part of salicylic acid. Coated aspirin products have made that side effect much less common, but for some the first warning of trouble is the diagnosis of an ulcer.

Millions of women were encouraged to take a variety of estrogen products for menopausal symptoms. Only in recent years has research determined that those estrogen pills came with an increased incidence of female cancers. Many of those women took estrogen for more than a decade, others for even longer periods. Must they all live now with the fear of developing a life-threatening illness?

Then there are the extremely powerful drugs that are prescribed for more serious conditions. Chemotherapy drugs attack cancer cells but also depress the body's healthy cell growth; steroids may do a terrific job of limiting the effects of asthma or rheumatoid arthritis in some patients, but what are the potential long-term effects of taking those drugs?

Those questions are still to be answered, but one thing is clear. You play an important role in your own health care, and you can take steps to ensure optimum health, whether or not you require prescription drugs.

## CAN YOU GET OFF PRESCRIPTION DRUGS?

Medication is a treatment option, not an absolute. Your physician's diagnosis of a medical concern or disease is only the first step in determining how you will be treated, managed, even cured.

Urgent care—what you get in the emergency room or from paramedics when you're having a heart attack or stroke, for instance—doesn't give you much of an opportunity to discuss a treatment plan with your caregivers. The goal at that moment is to save your life, prevent heart or brain damage, and get you stabilized.

But for most people, when your doctor says, "I'm going to give you a prescription," that should be when you ask for the information you need to participate actively in your care. Chapter 9 gave you a list of good questions to ask your physician and pharmacist about your prescribed medication. Another question may be "Is there anything I should be doing to help myself eventually get off this medication?"

Drugs for an infection, of course, have a time limit—usually a couple of weeks—and then you're done. By that time the medication should have done its job by wiping out the bacteria that caused the infection in the first place. But you may want to discuss drugs prescribed to help you manage a chronic condition, especially if they have side effects that could affect your health or lifestyle.

Let's take a look at common conditions, medication prescribed for them, and possible ways to lessen or alleviate your need for that medication. Note: *Always* work with your doctor with any medication changes. If, for instance, you take medication to manage type 2 diabetes and you then lose weight and cut sugar out of your diet, your doctor can let you know if you still need your medication or if it's time to decrease your dose.

## FOR HIGH CHOLESTEROL
## OR HIGH BLOOD PRESSURE

High blood pressure (hypertension) and high cholesterol are two of the most common health concerns in America, and the prescription drugs to treat them are some of the most profitable products any pharmaceutical company makes. Is there anything you can do to trim those profits?

### IMPROVE YOUR LIFESTYLE

You can start by "trimming" your own waistline and getting regular exercise. Your physician and other health-care professionals can advise you how to change some unhealthy habits. Those lifestyle changes, maintained over time, can make you a candidate for getting off your prescription medicine. For some people, however, their higher-than-healthy cholesterol or blood pressure doesn't respond to changes in diet or exercise, or not enough to eliminate the need for medication. But your doctor may be able to lower your dosage.

### TAKE OFF A FEW POUNDS

Many patients succeed in reducing their cholesterol or blood pressure through slow and steady weight loss (combined with healthy eating and exercise). The same is true about high blood pressure. For an obese person, losing even 10 percent of his or her body weight will usually reduce blood pressure to some extent. Coupled with a sensible exercise program and dietary changes that can help lower the numbers, modest weight loss is a great way to work toward less dependence on medication.

### PUMP UP THE MAGNESIUM

Recent studies suggest that magnesium may help regulate blood pressure. Diets that include lots of fruits and vegetables, which are good sources of potassium and magnesium, are generally linked to lower blood pressure. The widely reported DASH study (Dietary Approaches to Stop Hypertension) suggested that high blood pressure could be significantly lowered by a diet high in magnesium, potassium, and calcium, and low in sodium and fat. Another study examined the nutrition styles of more than thirty thousand male health professionals in the United States to discover the effect of diet on blood pressure. They found that a greater magnesium intake was associated with a lower risk of hypertension. With such convincing evidence, the Joint National Committee on Prevention, Detection, Evaluation, and Treatment of High Blood Pressure recommends maintaining an adequate magnesium intake to help prevent and manage high blood pressure.

### LIMIT YOUR SODIUM

Sodium reduction also appears to have a powerful effect on hypertension. The most recent report of the Joint National Committee notes that a diet with no more than 1,600 milligrams of sodium daily has effects "similar to single drug therapy." If your physician has prescribed hydrochlorothiazide to help reduce your blood pressure, and you also reduce your dietary sodium, you may be able to have your dosage decreased. The report goes on to say that if patients can achieve even better results if they commit to two lifestyle regimen changes (weight reduction in addition to sodium reduction, for instance).

## YOU CAN HELP AVOID TYPE 2 DIABETES

The National Institutes of Health trumpeted "Diet and Exercise Dramatically Delay Type 2 Diabetes" in an August 2001 press release. The report stated that the more than ten million Americans who are at risk for type 2 diabetes can "sharply lower their chances of getting the disease with diet and exercise," according to the findings of a major clinical trial, the Diabetes Prevention Program (DPP).

"In view of the rapidly rising rates of obesity and diabetes in America, this good news couldn't come at a better time," said Health and Human Services Secretary Tommy Thompson. "So many of our health problems can be avoided through diet, exercise and making sure we take care of ourselves." The study reported that those who made serious lifestyle changes reduced their risk by as much as 58 percent. This group committed to moderate physical activity such as walking for thirty minutes per day and lost 5 to 7 percent of their body weight.

Those who made healthy lifestyle changes did better than participants who took the oral diabetes drug metformin (Glucophage). The DPP also made a special effort to recruit members of minority groups who have a higher risk of developing type 2 diabetes—African Americans, Hispanic Americans, Asian Americans, Pacific Islanders, and Native Americans. The program also invited people known to be at high risk for other reasons—those over sixty years of age, women who had had gestational diabetes (during pregnancy), and anyone with a close relative who had the disease.

"Lifestyle intervention worked as well in men and women and in all the ethnic groups. It also worked well in people age sixty and older, who have a nearly 20 percent prevalence of diabetes, reducing the development of diabetes by 71 percent," said Dr. David Nathan of Massachusetts General Hospital in Boston.

The U.S. Department of Health and Human Services (HHS) publishes the statistics on this chronic disease, and the news isn't great: According to HHS, diabetes afflicts more than sixteen million people in the United States. It is the main cause of kidney failure, limb amputations, and new onset blindness in adults and a major cause of heart disease and stroke. Type 2 diabetes accounts for up to 95 percent of all diabetes cases. Most common in adults over age forty, type 2 diabetes affects 8 percent of the U.S. population age twenty and older. It is strongly associated with obesity (more than 80 percent of people with type 2 diabetes are overweight), inactivity, family history of diabetes, and racial or ethnic background. Compared to whites, black adults have a 60 percent higher rate of type 2 diabetes and Hispanic adults have a 90 percent higher rate.

Consult your physician for advice before starting an exercise program. Opt for a heart-healthy eating plan, and consider finding a support group to strengthen your resolve. A walking buddy will encourage you to exercise; a weight-loss partner can make it easier to make healthier choices.

## If You're Coping with Arthritis

The Arthritis Foundation (www. arthritis.org) offers helpful and up-to-date information about managing your arthritis symptoms with other therapies besides prescription medications. It offers excellent brochures about supplements, alternative therapies, exercise, and ways to work better with your doctor.

More than thirty-five million Americans are affected by osteoarthritis (OA), which can range from occasional mild pain and slightly swollen joints of the hands and feet to more debilitating weakness and disability. While at one time most medical professionals gave little credence to nutritional therapies, many now are satisfied that research into the use of vitamins and antioxidants has demonstrated their value. Vitamin C is widely recommended, as is making reasonable efforts to lose excess body weight, which stresses body joints, especially in knees and hips.

## GLUCOSAMINE AND CHONDROITIN

Jean Carper, who writes a popular health column for *USA Weekend*, described her own self-care and stated that she takes a daily supplement of glucosamine and chondroitin, which both relieves pain and can improve joint function in OA patients. She quotes a Belgian study that found the supplements safe and useful, and a spokesman for the Arthritis Foundation added that glucosamine and chondroitin performed equally well or better than traditional NSAIDS (non-steroidal anti-inflammatory drugs) like aspirin. Visit the Arthritis Foundation at www.arthritis.org/conditions/alttherapies/Glucosamine.asp for information regarding these supplements.

## SAM-E

Another supplement that has been widely studied is SAM-e, a natural sulfur compound that should be taken under medical supervision, according to Carper. This natural remedy, which has been very popular in Europe, began to be widely used in the past few years. An article in *Arthritis Today* noted that "Sammy" appears to cause fewer drug interactions or side effects than nonsteroidal anti-inflammatories such as aspirin and may also be useful for treating depression and fibromyalgia. Though many physicians are reserving judgment until more long-term studies are done, others are encouraging their patients to use it in modest amounts with careful oversight.

## FISH OIL

In the March 2003 issue of the *Annals of the Rheumatic Diseases*, rheumatoid arthritis patients in a small study in Sweden enjoyed reduced pain and less inflammation of joints after three months of eating a Mediterranean-style diet, which emphasizes legumes, fruits, vegetables, fish, and olive oil. Fish oil capsules, which are known to have an anti-inflammatory effect, are a widely recommended supplement for many rheumatoid arthritis patients. Reports that it helps to reduce swelling and to lessen pain and stiffness make it a popular supplement choice.

Treatments that show limited or little effect on symptoms, according to Carper, include MSM (methylsulfonylmethane) for osteoarthritis and cat's claw, a popular herbal, for rheumatoid arthritis. It's up to you to stay informed by visiting reliable arthritis Web sites such as www.arthritis.org for the results of ongoing studies.

## IF ALLERGIES ARE A PROBLEM

Many Americans suffer with the seasonal symptoms of various allergies, from pollen and dust mites to mold and animal dander. You can often manage allergic reactions to elements in your environment and reduce your dependence on medication, whether prescribed or over-the-counter.

Allergy Choices at www.allergychoices.com offers all kinds of good advice for coping with different sensitivities. These suggestions include:

- Removing carpeting in favor of hard surface floors
- Using hot water heat instead of "forced air"
- Reducing humidity to between 35 and 40 percent
- Decorating with window shades instead of Venetian blinds to avoid dust accumulation
- Limiting the number of indoor plants you have, and if your allergies are severe, choosing an artificial Christmas tree over a live one

Although recommendations vary according to what you're allergic to (mold, dust, pet dander, and so on), you can reduce or eliminate allergens room by room in your house. For instance, an exhaust fan in the kitchen and regularly emptying the pan under your refrigerator's defrosting unit can help decrease mold levels. Simply keeping a pet out of the bedroom can greatly help the allergic member of your family. Keep well hydrated, because the amount of water in your body's tissues affects your histamine production. Use and frequently replace air filters in your house (use a face mask or ask a nonallergic person to do this job). For more resources on allergies, try the American Academy of Allergy, Asthma and Immunology Web site (www.aaaai.org). You can find publications and information sheets on such items as asthma triggers, food allergies, and environmental controls.

The list of suggestions is too long to cover here, but with some extra effort you can make your home a "haven" from allergens. Your attention to these kinds of details can be your first line of defense when it comes to avoiding allergy symptoms and needing less medication.

## IF YOU'RE ACHING WITH ACID REFLUX

With acid reflux disease (also called GERD, gastroesophageal reflux disease) your esophagus—the tube stretching from your throat to your stomach—becomes irritated or inflamed because acid backs up from your stomach. Your swallowed food travels down the esophagus to the stomach, which produces hydrochloric acid to help in digestion. Your stomach lining isn't damaged by the acid, but your esophagus can be when the ring of muscle at its bottom, the lower esophageal sphincter, weakens or relaxes between swallows to allow stomach acid to flow upward.

What can you do if you experience acid reflux symptoms but want to rely less on prescription medication? Here are some possibilities:

- Make some lifestyle changes that can help: Lose weight, eliminate alcohol and cigarettes, and work to correct poor posture (slouching).

- Tackle your diet: Avoid or reduce your intake of fatty and fried foods, chocolate, garlic and onions, drinks with caffeine, acidic foods (citrus fruits, tomatoes), spicy foods, and anything with mint flavoring.

- Change *how* you eat: Stop eating large meals, don't lie down after eating, and stop eating at least three hours before bedtime.

- Elevate the head of your bed by putting blocks under the box spring. Lift it at least six to eight inches.

- Avoid over-the-counter pain relievers such as aspirin and ibuprofen (Advil, Motrin), which can cause reflux symptoms in some people.

- Don't exercise on a full stomach or plan activities that require a lot of bending over. Gravity can work against you with acid reflux disease.

If these self-care options don't eliminate symptoms, don't delay in speaking to your physician about medication. Acid reflux can lead to dangerous health complications and should be treated without fail.

## IF YOU'RE IN THE MIDST OF MENOPAUSE

Now that estrogen therapy is considered more risky than in the past, many post-menopausal women and their physicians are opting for other symptom relief.

Troublesome menopausal symptoms include hot flashes, which are an annoyance, but more crucial are the vaginal dryness and the lack of estrogen that helps keep bones healthy. Don't hesitate to talk to your doctor about your concerns and to ask for guidance. Here is just a sampling of some of the tips that may help.

### PUMP UP THE CALCIUM

Nutritional advice from the American College of Obstetricians and Gynecologists for women facing menopause centers on a healthy diet, with a variety of foods to ensure you get all the nutrients you require. Your best bet is a low-fat, low-cholesterol regime that includes enough calcium to keep your bones strong. Current recommendations are 1,000 milligrams per day for women getting hormone replacement therapy and 1,500 milligrams if they are not. If you're not consuming enough calcium, talk to your doctor about whether supplements are right for you and which ones are best for delaying bone loss. You also need vitamin D for bone health, which you can get from fortified milk or from as little as fifteen minutes of daily exposure to the sun.

### INCREASE YOUR EXERCISE

Exercise is highly recommended, especially weight-bearing exercise to strengthen bones. Many women in their fifties and beyond are choosing to add weight training to their exercise programs, and many report an increase in metabolism, better circulation, and an overall feeling of well-being.

### TURN TO PHYTOESTROGENS

Increase your intake of foods that contain phytoestrogens, including soy, and healthy grains, including oats, wheat, brown rice, tofu, almonds, cashews, and fresh fruits and vegetables.

## CONSIDER VITAMINS AND MINERALS

Vitamin E has been shown to reduce night sweats and hot flashes in some women; magnesium improves calcium absorption; vitamin C helps the absorption of E.

## AVOID PHOSPHORUS

Other studies suggest reducing caffeine and drinking fewer carbonated beverages, which contain phosphorus and can contribute to bone loss.

# KEEP YOUR HEART HEALTHY

Much of the advice offered throughout this chapter is also valid for anyone concerned about preventing heart disease. Priorities include losing excess weight by eating a healthy diet; getting regular, heart-pumping exercise; reducing your cholesterol count to a healthy number; and lowering your blood pressure to a healthy pair of numbers.

There's a whole new category for blood-pressure checkups called "pre-hypertension." It describes blood pressure levels at 120–139 (systolic) and 80-89 (diastolic) as potentially dangerous.

In the past, we used to think 140 over 90 was okay. Today, the American Heart Association (AHA) has lowered the numbers for what constitutes a "healthy heart." Your cholesterol numbers are also vitally important. Check your personal numbers with these charts provided by the AHA:

| Classification | Systolic | Diastolic |
|---|---|---|
| Normal | 120 | 80 |
| Pre-Hypertension | 120–139 | 80–89 |
| Stage 1 Hypertension | 140–159 | 90–99 |
| State 2 Hypertension | 160 | 100 |

For people over fifty, systolic is more important than distolic.

The soft waxy substance found in the lipids (fats) in your blood stream is your cholesterol. If the lipid levels get too high, you are in danger of clogging your blood vessels. It's recommended that everyone over the age of twenty have a lipoprotein (cholesterol) test every five years. (It should be tested more often, if abnormalities are noted.) Your doctor interprets the various cholesterol classifications and the numbers involved. The quotations will cover: Total Cholesterol, HDL ("good") Cholesterol, and LDL ("bad") Cholesterol. High levels of LDL should be reduced and low HDL levels should be elevated. Total cholesterol should be kept at normal levels. This AHA chart gives you an idea of what to aim for:

| Levels | Category |
| --- | --- |
| *HDL* | |
| Less than 40 mg/dl | Too Low (the higher the better) |
| *LDL* | |
| Less than 100 mg/dl | Optimal |
| 100–129 mg/dl | Near Optimal |
| 130–159 mg/dl | Borderline High |
| 160–189 mg/dl | High |
| 190 mg/dl and above | Very High |
| *Total Cholesterol* | |
| Less than 200 mg/dl | Desirable |
| 200–239 mg/dl | Borderline High |
| 240 mg/dl | Too High |

Other strategies can demonstrably reduce the likelihood of your developing a heart ailment. These include:

## QUITTING SMOKING

Cities such as New York have made it harder and harder to find a place to smoke, now that offices, bars, and restaurants are off-limits. There's never been a better time to stop smoking. Many companies offer programs for their employees who want to quit—take advantage of whatever is available to do it now. Your heart will thank you for it.

## Triglycerides

Triglycerides are the most common kind of fat in the body. Along with your cholesterol checkup, your physician will want to take a look at your triglyceride levels. Many people who have heart disease or diabetes have high triglycerides.

| Trygliceride Level | Category |
| --- | --- |
| Less than 150 mg/dl | Normal |
| 150–199 mg/dl | Borderline High |
| 200–499 mg/dl | High |
| 500 mg/dl and above | Very High |

### LOWERING ALCOHOL INTAKE

Current research suggests that limiting consumption of alcohol will pay off big when it comes to your overall health.

### REDUCING STRESS

For optimum health, you need to examine your "stress style." If you overreact to frustration or family issues, you may be making yourself sick. If you frequently experience anger and hostility at home or at work, you are in real danger—and you are the only one who can choose to change how you respond to these triggers. Try to choose safe outlets for your frustration, make lifestyle changes, or ask for help from a counselor.

As you can see, you're not completely at the mercy of the pharmaceutical companies. You can use many strategies to strengthen your resistance to disease, improve your overall physical condition, and lower your risk of developing more serious illnesses. You may not be able to eliminate the need for any prescription medication, but with these techniques, you may succeed in requiring a lot less.

Good luck!

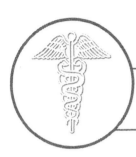

EIGHTEEN

# THE NEXT AMERICAN REVOLUTION

W hen the American colonists decided to sever the ties with England nearly two and a half centuries ago, the decision had as much to do with economics as with a desire for national independence. They resented paying excessive prices set by their English overlords. They began with boycotts—but they were finally willing to fight a war for their freedom from financial enslavement.

Today, American citizens are rebelling against the same kinds of economic unfairness, angry about being overcharged for products that American companies market to the rest of the world at lower prices. A *New York Times* cover story reveals that American college students are paying twice as much as British students for the very same, U.S.-published textbooks. The companies insist they wouldn't be able to sell the books abroad unless they carried lower prices. But a representative of the National Association of College Stores calls it "price-gouging of the American public generally and college students in particular." (This publishers' practice remarkably mirrors the excessive profit-taking by pharmaceutical companies at the expense of American consumers, many of them elderly, poor, and chronically ill.)

## SHOULD HEALTH CARE BE
## A FOR-PROFIT BUSINESS?

While national debate continues about the high price of prescription drugs, an ABC News/*Washington Post* poll found that 70 percent of all Americans said it should be legal for Americans to buy prescription drugs outside the United States, and one in eight have done it. Fifty-four percent are dissatisfied with the overall quality of health care in the United States—10 percent more than a similar poll found in 2000.

The poll also asked about other health-care concerns. Sixty percent admitted they were worried about being able to afford health insurance, and one in six had no health insurance. More than 15 percent of Americans are currently uninsured, and more than half of those who are insured worry about losing their health insurance if they were to lose their jobs.

Perhaps the most significant response in the poll and by a two-to-one margin (62 percent to 32 percent), Americans said they would prefer a universal health-care system that would provide coverage to everyone under a government program, as opposed to the employer-based system we have now. Only a year ago, fewer than half of those polled favored the idea of a national health coverage program.

Congress continues to work on legislation providing improved Medicare drug coverage and other laws designed to allow Americans to purchase cheaper drugs from across the border. "The high cost of prescription drugs ends up being just as harmful as the diseases people are fighting," said Representative Jo Ann Emerson of Missouri, a cosponsor of the prescription drug reimportation measure.

The price of prescription drugs keeps going up and up year after year. If you need to take three, four, or five different drugs each month, you are probably spending much too high a percentage of your income on medicine. Taking those medicines is not a luxury, like dining at a four-star restaurant. It's a necessity for maintaining the quality of life, for sustaining life itself.

## TAMING THE PHARMACEUTICAL COMPANIES

So what can we do? A growing political movement is aimed at taming the pharmaceutical companies. People are letting their state lawmakers know how angry they feel about being priced out of the prescription drug market. Some state governments are even heeding the call by setting up bulk-buying drug purchase plans to avoid overpaying for medicine. So countering the big-money lobbying organized by the pharmaceutical companies *can* work. It's just that up to now, not enough have joined to fight back. But the scent of revolution is in the air.

A telltale sign that political winds might be changing is the fact that thousands of seniors are traveling to Canada and Mexico in bus and car caravans to buy their prescriptions at half the price they pay in the United States. But why should these elder Americans, citizens of the richest, most powerful country in the world, have to head for another country to buy the same American-made prescription drugs they'd pay double for if they bought them here? The companies keep raising prices and nobody has been willing to say "Whoa." At least, not until recently.

The companies say that unless consumers pay these high prices, they'll be unable to fund research to discover new drugs. It's true that pharmaceutical research costs a lot and may take years before paying off. But, taxpayers are also funding huge executive salaries. Here's what the Families USA report, "Profiting from Pain," listed as three of the ten highest paid executives' 2001 annual compensation (exclusive of unexercised stock options):

- C. A. Heimbold Jr., former chairman and CEO, Bristol-Myers Squibb Co., $74,890,918

- John R. Stafford, chairman, Wyeth, $40,521,011

- William C. Steere, former chairman, Pfizer, Inc., $28,264,282

The pharmaceutical industry spends millions of dollars annually to wine and dine and otherwise try to influence members of Congress and state legislators. This powerful lobby, called PhRMA, has a very specific agenda: to shoot down any legislation designed to limit their profits.

They're all for having prescription drug benefits as part of Medicare, but only as long as there is no attempt by the federal government to put a cap on prices—even though the federal government would be putting up the money. PhRMA lobbyists have seen the future as scripted in some of the New England states, and it doesn't look good for them. They come up big losers when local governments use their bulk purchasing power to cap drug prices for the citizens of their states.

## DEMOCRACY DEMANDS ACTION

Don't throw up your hands and mutter: "Politics—what can you do?" As an individual, your power is modest. But as a member of a national organization, you can pay your dues and join the fray. If you or your spouse is age fifty or older, you can join your local AARP chapter. It's listed in the phone book, or visit www.aarp.org. AARP has been fighting for price controls on prescription drugs ever since the fight began.

Visit the Web site of the Public Citizen organization, based in Washington, D.C., at www.publiccitizen.org to keep up with what's going on in Congress about prescription drugs, reimportation from Canada, and other related issues.

Another good political action group is The National Center to Preserve Social Security and Medicare. This organization primarily lobbies members of Congress to legislate Medicare prescription benefits. Membership dues are only $10 a year. For more information, call (800) 966-1935. It's a real bargain if you'd like to get into the Medicare lobbying business.

### Direct Dial Congress

The National Center to Preserve Social Security and Medicare has set up a direct line to your two senators and your member of Congress. Just dial (800) 998-0180 to get instructions that tell you how to be connected directly to their offices. Let them hear what you have to say about prescription drug prices. Call today!

## BANKING ON YOUR BUSINESS

That's the political side of the prescription drug wars. Now let's look at the business side. When it comes to buying smart, consider yourself a small business owner concerned about the bottom line. You must buy supplies to keep your business (that is, you and your family) going. And one of your major expenditures in the business plan (family budget) is medication.

You might want to set up a filing cabinet section or a desk drawer to collect and keep the information you find about getting the best prices for your prescription drugs. Throughout this book, you will find helpful Web sites. This is a good list to clip and file for future reference:

- American Pharmacists Association (APA) and the National Association of Boards of Pharmacy Web site, www.pharmacist.com, sells a number of valuable publications such as, *Medication Errors* and the *Handbook of Prescription Drugs*.

- The APA has another Web site, www.pharmacyandyou.org, that provides in-depth information about pharmacists.

- The National Council on Patient Information and Education Web site, www.bemedwise.org, provides much useful information such as, tips, brochures, and kits that help you understand things like drug interactions, over-the-counter drugs, and reading drug labels.

- The National Council on Patient Information and Education Web site, www.talkaboutrx.org, a sister site to Be MedWise, provides information on such topics as, Anthrax, antibiotics, dietary supplements and herbal medicines, online purchasing, and questions to ask about prescriptions.

- The Food and Drug Administration Web site, www.FDA.gov, offers all the information you could possibly want on drugs, including buying drugs on the Internet.

- The National Council on Aging Web site, www.benefitscheckup.org, has a section called "BenefitsCheckUpRX" that directs you to fill out a questionnaire, after which you are shown a list of potential prescription discount benefits.

- The National Association of Boards of Pharmacy Web site, www.nabp.net, provides information about pharmacies and pharmacists. They have a list of acceptable online pharmacies under the heading VIPPS.

## Summing Up

By changing how you view yourself, and by recognizing that you're both a business owner and a political lobbyist, you can begin to reclaim your power when paying for your medicines.

You now have a wealth of information about the best ways to get the best prices for the drugs you need. You know what to look for and the questions to ask about your drugs so you can be sure of your safety and protect the health of your family.

That's what it is all about: your money and your health. Two more important elements of a good life that together add up to a winning equation. In the words of an old Spanish banquet toast: *Salud, pesetas, y amor, y tiempo para gosarlo.* Translation: Health, money, and love, and time to enjoy it.

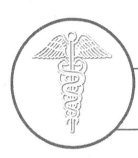

# APPENDIX

# SMART MEDICINE RESOURCE CENTER

Throughout the book, you have seen some resources cited: Web sites and phone numbers. We've pulled them together here, along with some new listings. You might want to tear this out and put it in your files. Basically, they fall under three broad categories: government, nonprofits, and commercial.

## GOVERNMENT

### THE FOOD AND DRUG ADMINISTRATION (FDA)

www.fda.gov

This site is exhaustive in the information it provides on drugs. There is even a section on the ins and outs of buying drugs online.

### NATIONAL CENTER FOR COMPLEMENTARY AND ALTERNATIVE MEDICINE

www.nccam.nih.gov

A companion website to the FDA, this site includes publications, information for researchers, frequently asked questions, and links to other CAM-related resources.

It provides health information, including Alerts and Advisories and links to other organizations.

## The Department of Veterans Affairs (VA)

www.VA.gov – 877-222-VETS

If you have ever served in the armed forces, you should check out the VA's website to see if you might qualify for medical benefits, including prescription and non-prescription drugs.

## Nonprofits

### Institute for Safe Medication Practices

www.ismp.org

The Institute for Safe Medication Practices (ISMP) is a nonprofit organization that works closely with health-care practitioners and institutions, regulatory agencies, professional organizations and the pharmaceutical industry to provide education about adverse drug events and their prevention.

### American Pharmacists Association

www.pharmacyandyou.org

It provides in-depth information about pharmacists, everything from facts about pharmacists and how to get the most out of your pharmacist to consumer tips and drug interactions.

### The Alliance for Retired Americans

www.retiredamericans.org

It's a way for retired union members and others to make their voices heard. They provide news about getting better prescription prices through political and legal action. With membership, it provides many benefits, including affordable health insurance.

## AMERICAN ASSOCIATION OF RETIRED PERSONS (AARP)

www.aarp.org

Here you can find out about the latest legislations, information on everything from prescription drugs and insurance to eating well and managing stress.

## THE NATIONAL CONSUMERS LEAGUE

www.nclnet.org

NCL provides you with the consumer's perspective on concerns including, among other things, medication information.

## NATIONAL COUNCIL ON AGING

www.ncoa.org

This provides information on what prescription drug benefits you may qualify to receive.

## NATIONAL COUNCIL ON PATIENT

www.talkaboutrx.org

A sister site to BeMedWise.com, it has information on Information and Education prescription and over-the-counter drugs, dietary supplements, herbal medicines, and online purchasing. It also provides a list of questions to ask your physician and pharmacist.

## MINNESOTA SENIOR FEDERATION

www.mnseniors.org

A grassroots advocacy organization for seniors, this site has information on how to import prescription drugs from Canada through the organization's special relationships with Canadian pharmacies. The service is not limited to Minnesota residents.

## RxAssist

www.rxassist.org

RxAssist is a national program supported by the Robert Wood Johnson Foundation. This Web site provides a list of state programs, a comparative chart of thje drug companies discount cards, and allows you to search by drug, drug class, or company to find different discount programs available.

## COMMERCIAL

### National Association of Boards of Pharmacy

www.nabp.net

They have a list of VIPPS certified online pharmacies located in the U.S. and Canada (and some in Mexico). To be VIPPS certified pharmacies must comply with the licensing and inspection requirements of their state and those in which the dispense drugs.

### Rx List

www.rxlist.com

You can access the Internet Drug List with a link to order prescriptions at wholesale prices. You can't purchase the drugs at this site but there's a link to a certified VIPPS pharmacy you can reach through an online drugstore link where you are put in touch with a licensed pharmacist.

### NeedyMeds.com

www.needymeds.com

For information on how to get free drugs for income-challenged patients, go to this site. It provides a list of 266 assistance programs; applications for the different assistance programs available through pharmaceutical companies; a list of over 1,300 generic drugs; and more.

## Be MedWise

www.bemedwise.com

National Council on Patient Information and Education's Web site that provides much useful information such as, tips, brochures, and kits that help you understand things like drug interactions, over-the-counter drugs, and reading drug labels.

## Senior Care Pharmacists

www.seniorcarepharmacist.com

They are members of the American Society of Consultant Pharmacists and the Web site has information on how to use medicines wisely to avoid interactions and other problems.

## AffordableRX

www.affordablerx.com

This is a great site for information on buying drugs from Canada.

## AARP Health Care Options

www.aarphealthcare.com

You can find out about the association's supplemental medical insurance. Some chapters have access to their states' bulk-purchase, discount drugs.

## The Medicine Program

www.themedicineprogram.com

This organization was established by volunteers dedicated to alleviating the plight of an ever increasing number of patients who cannot afford their prescription medication.

## United Benefit Advisors

www.benefits.com

This site provides business owners with solutions to employee benefit needs.

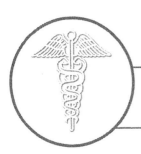

# Index

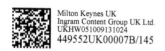